Men's Fitness magazine

COMPLETE TRAINING GUIDE

By Pete Muir

Photography **Tom Miles**
Design **Marco Crisari**
Illustrations **Roger Gorringe**
Subeditor **Juliet Giles**
Model **Toby Rowland @ Nevs**

With thanks to

FitnessFirst

www.fitnessfirst.co.uk

For more information on *Men's Fitness* magazine, go to mensfitnessmagazine.co.uk.
To subscribe call 0844 844 0081.

Dennis Publishing

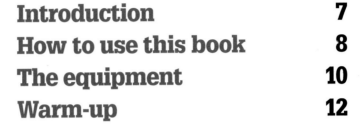

Contents

Introduction   **7**

How to use this book   **8**

The equipment   **10**

Warm-up   **12**

Arms   **15**

Abs   **45**

Back   **71**

Chest   **91**

Legs   **109**

Shoulders   **133**

Total body   **151**

Stretching   **162**

How to build a workout   **164**

Tips on working out   **174**

The cardio question   **176**

Chart your progress   **178**

Nutrition   **181**

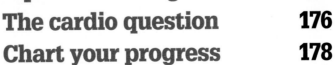

Here we go

Welcome to the *Complete Training Guide*. Brought to you by the people who create *Men's Fitness* magazine every month, this is the ultimate reference guide for anyone who wants to change their body shape.

For many years it has been proven that the best way to achieve this is through weight training, and this guide provides everything you need to know about training with weights safely and effectively. Put simply, by working your muscles against a resistance you create tiny tears in your muscle fibres that heal bigger and stronger than they were before. Building muscle is also an effective way of burning fat because your body is obliged to burn up calories from your fat stores simply by sustaining the extra muscle you carry. Of course, this doesn't mean you can live off pizzas and expect to have the body of an Olympic athlete, but we will discuss the best things to eat at the end of the book.

WHAT'S IN THE *COMPLETE TRAINING GUIDE*?

Inside you'll find demonstrations and explanations for more than 240 of the best exercises to build every part of your body. Why so many? Well, most men stick to the same few exercises every time they go to the gym – the ones they know and are comfortable with – however experience shows that people who always do the same exercises soon stop adding new muscle because their bodies have adapted to their routines and are no longer stimulated.

To keep adding muscle you need continually to change your workout routine to keep your body stimulated. That's why we have provided you with enough exercises for you to change your workout frequently without ever doing the same routine twice. This has the additional benefit of keeping your brain stimulated, so you don't get bored and give up on your training regime after only a few weeks.

WHAT ELSE WILL YOU FIND?

As well as the main exercises, you'll find comprehensive warm-up and stretching routines, plus details on equipment and how to build a workout. There's also information on eating properly to gain muscle without putting on fat.

This guide will teach you the principles of effective weight training and provide you with all the ammunition you need to start your own training regime with confidence and get the body you've always wanted.

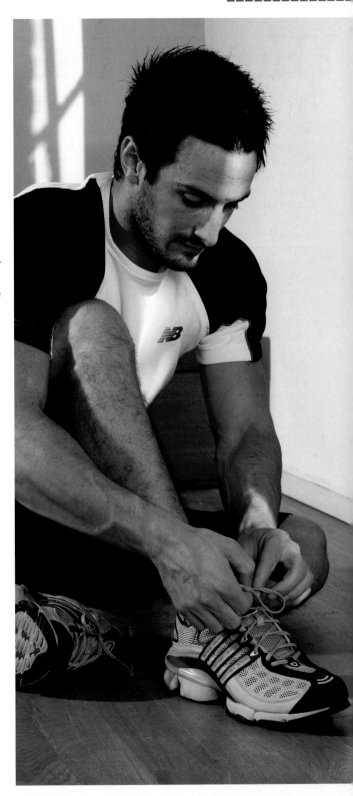

How to use this book

The *Complete Training Guide* is perfect for beginners or experienced weight trainers alike. If you are familiar with gyms, have trained with weights before and know your goals, then you can simply use this book as a reference guide to the best exercises for each muscle group. If you are new to training, you'll find tips and advice on building a workout regime, training effectively and eating to increase muscle.

We start with an introduction to the main items of equipment you'll be using (p10) and then provide you with the perfect pre-workout warm-up (p12). Then we move on to the exercises themselves, which make up the bulk of the *Complete Training Guide*.

We've divided the exercises by body part. On page 15 you'll find a chapter dedicated to exercises that build muscles in the arms. This is followed by chapters on abs, back, chest, legs, shoulders and 'total body'. Of course, many exercises work muscles in several parts of the body at once, but we have usually given only the target muscle for each exercise. For example, the bench press (p94) is in the 'chest' chapter even though the exercise also trains muscles in the arms, shoulders and torso. With more than 600 muscles in the human body, we thought it best that each exercise only mentions the muscles you are targeting specifically.

On each spread we've demonstrated one main move, and then offered three 'variations'. The main moves are classic exercises that should be in every man's repertoire, and the variations ensure you always have an alternative when you need to perk up your training.

BUILDING A WORKOUT

After the exercise demonstrations, we provide details on how to arrange the exercises into workouts for the best results (p164). Most weight-training manuals give you a specific workout plan to follow, but this means that those books' usefulness comes to an end once you have completed the plan after a few weeks. Instead, we believe it is better to explain the basic principles behind effective workouts so that you can create your own and keep changing your workouts every few weeks.

From page 167 we outline seven different training principles and give examples of workouts that you can use as templates to create your own. We also offer tips to make each workout more effective (p174) and explain how to chart your progress over the weeks (p178).

EAT AND BE MERRY

At the end of this guide (p181) we'll tell you about what to eat and when to eat it, to ensure that your workouts are properly fuelled. We've also given you a one-week meal plan that provides the right combination of carbohydrates, protein, fats and vitamins to keep you healthy and build new muscle.

With everything that's in it, the *Complete Training Guide* is the most comprehensive weight training manual you can buy. We hope you enjoy it.

Advice for beginners

If you are new to exercising here are a few things to think about before you get started:
● Check with your GP before beginning any exercise regime, especially if you have a history of heart trouble.
● Always warm up properly before doing any serious exercise (see p12). This will help to prevent aches and strains occurring.
● If you feel pain at any time during your workout, stop immediately. Don't be tempted to work through the pain or you could do serious damage to muscles, joints or tendons.
● Maintain perfect form for every repetition (rep) of every exercise. Each exercise in this book comes with detailed notes on form, and most gyms have fitness experts who will be happy to help if you are still unsure about an exercise.
● Pick a weight you can manage easily the first time you perform any lifting exercise. This way you can concentrate on performing the exercise perfectly, and then you can build up the weight over time. Leave your ego at the door – choosing a weight that's too heavy for you is the fastest way to cut your training short through injury.
● You have hit 'failure' when you can't complete another rep of an exercise without breaking good form. So, if your training plan suggests you should perform each exercise 'to failure', it means you should stop when you can't lift a weight with perfect form, not when you can't lift the weight at all.
● In many of the form guides throughout this book you will see instructions saying 'brace your core

A few training myths busted

1 'Weight training will make me look overly bulky; I just want to tone up'
No-one has ever woken up after a weight training session to discover that they've turned into Arnold Schwarzenegger overnight. Weight training will increase muscle size, but gaining massive bulk takes years (and in many cases illegal steroids) so don't worry about sudden body changes.

Also, 'toning' is one of those terms that means nothing. If you want to tone up, what you are really saying is you want to build muscle and lose fat to look more defined, and that's exactly what this book is all about.

2 'Doing sit-ups will help me lose fat from my belly'
Sorry, you cannot lose fat from a specific part of your body. You can just lose fat generally, and the best way to do that is through proper diet and calorie-burning exercises. Sit-ups use very few muscles, and so burn very few calories, which makes them rubbish at getting rid of belly fat.

3 'More training equals bigger muscles'
Not quite true. You need to do the right amount of training to get the best results (find out more on p164). Any more is at best unnecessary, and at worst counter-productive. Doing too many weight training sessions in a week, or taking too much time for each session, can quickly lead to over-training, which can see you losing muscle instead of gaining it, and can lead to stress injuries.

4 'Aerobic exercise is best for fat loss and definition'
Aerobic exercise, such as running or cycling, is a great way of burning calories and improving heart and lung function, but often it can lead to a break down in muscle tissue as well. The best way to strip away fat is through a combination of weight training and cardiovascular exercise, done at the right times and right intensities. We will look more closely at cardio training on p176.

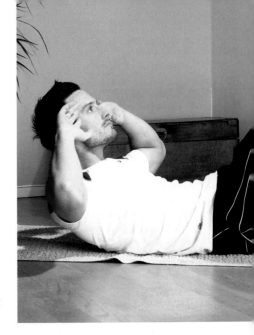

5 'I can re-shape my muscles by doing specific exercises'
Unfortunately, no. The shape of your muscles is decided purely by genetics. You can change the size of your muscles but not their shape.

6 'By doing weight training I can turn fat into muscle'
Fat and muscle are two entirely different tissues, and you cannot turn one into the other. If, through a combination of sitting on the sofa and eating pizzas, you allow your muscles to wither and fat to accumulate, it may seem as though your muscles have become fat, but it's not the case.

7 'The same training regime will have the same results for everybody'
Different people have different genetic make-up. Some people are naturally tall and thin (ectomorph), some are short and round (endomorph) and some are somewhere in between (mesomorph). If you are fortunate enough to be a mesomorph, you will find it easier to increase muscle mass than the ectomorph, and endomorphs will have a tougher time losing fat than the other two, but everyone can still improve their overall body shape by following the advice in this book.

muscles' or 'hold your core tight'. This means that you should contract the muscles around your midriff – especially your abdominals – to stabilise your spine while doing lifts.

To do this, start by ensuring that you are standing or sitting up straight with your hips in line with your torso. Now imagine that someone is about to punch you in the stomach and you have to tense your abdominal muscles to take the blow. You need to maintain that contraction throughout the move to protect your lower back from muscle strains.

● If you don't want to look like a beginner in the gym, remember a few basic points of gym etiquette. Always return any equipment to its place after using it, and don't hog equipment for too long. Wipe your sweat off machines, mats or benches after using them – gyms usually provide paper towels for this purpose. If someone is using the equipment you want, ask to 'work in' with them, which means you take turns doing a set of exercises while the other one rests.

● For more advice on training, plus detailed workouts and eating plans, see *Men's Fitness* magazine every month. Go to mensfitnessmagazine. co.uk for more details.

Tools of the trade

Everything you need for the perfect workout

Whenever you walk into a gym, there's always a dazzling array of equipment, much of it looking like it wouldn't be out of place in a medieval torture dungeon, but nearly all of it does the same job – providing resistance for your muscles to work against.

The equipment in a weights room can usually be split into two types: free weights and machines. Free weights include dumb-bells and barbells, and are called 'free' because you are not restricted as to how you use them. Most machines, by contrast, can only be used in one way and are designed to target a specific muscle group.

When you're performing the exercises found in this guide, the majority of the equipment you'll use will fall into the 'free-weight' category.

WHY NO MACHINES?

Machines can be extremely useful if you are starting a weights routine for the first time and are unsure of which exercises to perform. They lock your body into a particular plane of motion, and that helps to prevent you from injuring yourself. On the other hand, machines also prevent you from lifting weights naturally – you have to follow the path set by the machine, not your own natural path – so you won't be able to achieve the same muscle gains as you would be able to with free weights.

Also machines remove the need for you to stabilise your core muscles while performing lifts, so you may increase the strength of particular muscles, but you won't train your body to perform as a single, efficient unit.

Even if you start training with machines when you first join a gym, you should aim to move on to the free weights after a few weeks.

WHAT IF I DON'T HAVE A GYM?

Many of the items of equipment here can be bought for home use. If money is tight, you're best buying a set of adjustable dumb-bells and a Swiss ball. With just these two items you can perform hundreds of different exercises for every part of your body.

DUMB-BELLS
The main advantage of dumb-bells is that they work both sides of your body independently and allow for a natural range of movement in any exercise.

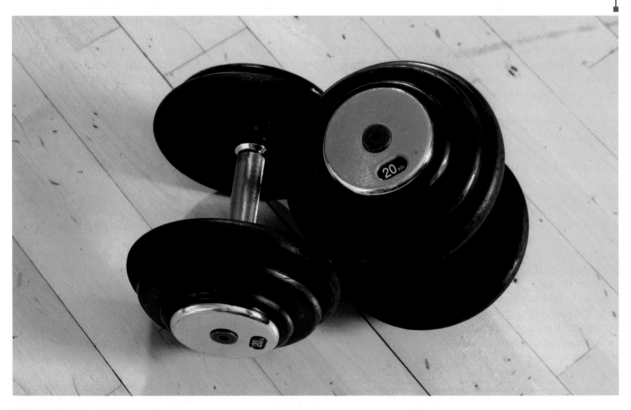

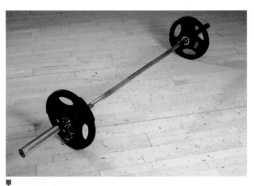

BARBELL
The bar allows you to lift heavy weights, so is great for building muscle mass, but is slightly more restrictive than dumb-bells in terms of range of movement.

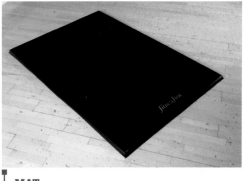

MAT
Vital for floor exercises such as crunches where you need to protect your spine.

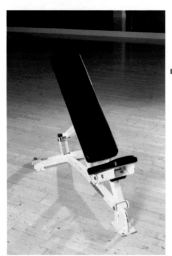

BENCH
A good bench should be rock solid, long enough to support your hips and head, and preferably be adjustable so you can use it flat or at an angle.

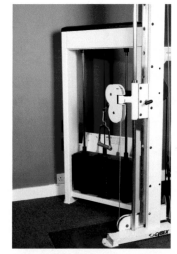

CABLE MACHINE
With a cable the resistance remains constant, regardless of the exercise you do. For example, if you do biceps curls with a barbell the resistance drops off as you near the top of the move. Not so with a cable curl.

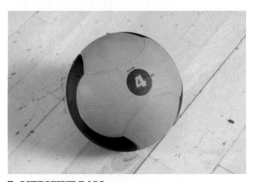

MEDICINE BALL
The advantage of a medicine ball is that you can drop it without smashing chunks out of the floor. This makes it good for the kind of dynamic moves that are replicated in sports.

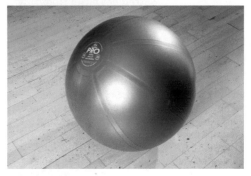

SWISS BALL
The Swiss ball adds an element of wobble to exercises, so it's great for training your core muscles – the ones around your trunk that help to stabilise your spine.

Get ready for action

Before every workout do this warm-up routine to prepare your muscles

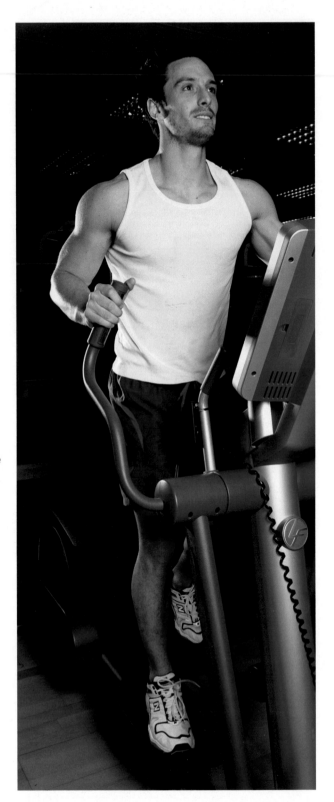

Spending ten or 15 minutes doing a warm-up before your workout can seem like valuable time wasted, but it's vital if you don't want to waste days laid up at home with damaged muscles or ligaments.

The purpose of a warm-up is simple: to raise your core temperature and prepare your muscles for the work to come. By doing some light cardiovascular exercise – such as running, cycling or rowing – you make your heart beat faster, which pumps oxygen and nutrients to your muscles and elevates your body's temperature. Warm muscles are more elastic, so you can work them through a greater range of motion with less chance of injury.

Once you've done the cardio warm-up, you should then move onto targeting the muscles directly with dynamic stretches. These will help to further increase the temperature of your muscles, stretch them gently and get them ready for heavy lifting. Dynamic stretches differ from static stretches (see p162) because you are moving continuously, placing the muscle under tension a little bit more with each repetition, thereby preparing the muscles, joints and nerves for the actions they are about to perform.

Once you begin your workout it makes sense to do your first set of each lift with a light weight, so that you further prepare the specific muscles and tendons you are targeting for heavier weights in the following sets.

WARM-UP: CARDIO

Begin with ten minutes of gentle cardio such as running, rowing, cycling or cross-training. By the end you should be sweating gently and puffing, but not out of breath. You don't want to burn out before your workout begins!

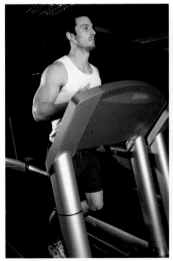
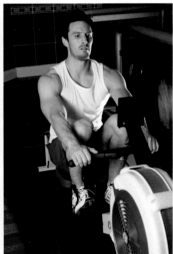
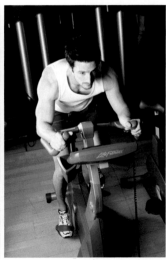

WARM-UP: DYNAMIC STRETCHES

Do ten repetitions of each of the following exercises, alternating sides with each rep where appropriate. Start gently and aim to increase the range of motion with each rep.

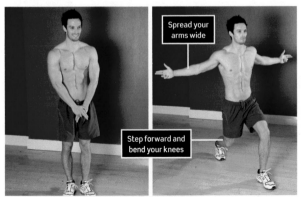

Spread your arms wide

Step forward and bend your knees

1. LUNGE WITH REVERSE FLYE

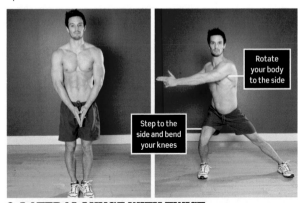

Rotate your body to the side

Step to the side and bend your knees

2. LATERAL LUNGE WITH TWIST

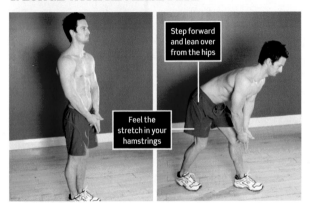

Step forward and lean over from the hips

Feel the stretch in your hamstrings

3. ALTERNATING SPLIT DEADLIFT

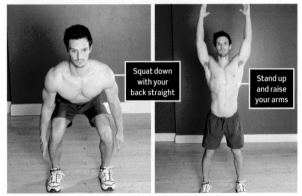

Squat down with your back straight

Stand up and raise your arms

4. SQUAT-TO-OVERHEAD REACH

ARMS

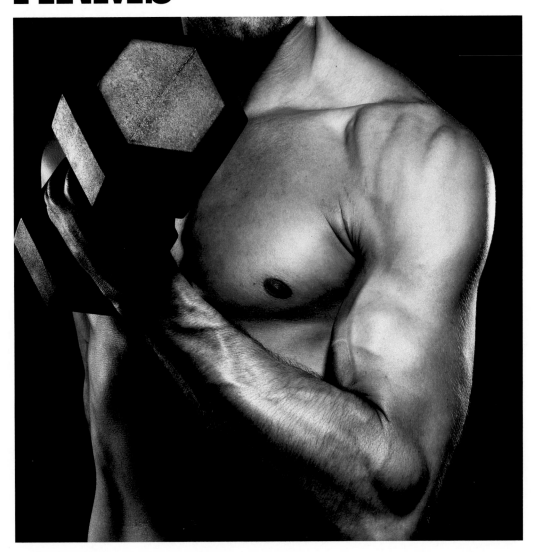

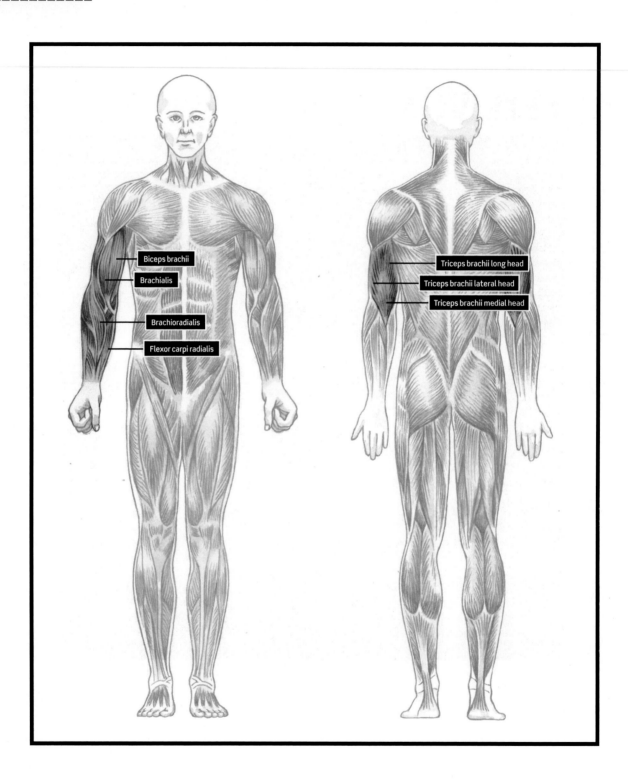

Biceps brachii

Brachialis

Brachioradialis

Flexor carpi radialis

Triceps brachii long head

Triceps brachii lateral head

Triceps brachii medial head

ARMS

The biceps come high up the list of glamour muscles for most men. It's the muscle you flex when you want to show off your muscles. Go into any gym and you'll see rows of men curling barbells in an attempt to build bulging biceps. Yet the biceps are among the smaller muscles in the body, and they aren't even the biggest muscles in your arms.

Your triceps make up about two thirds of your upper arm muscle mass and, as the name suggests, they are made up of three different muscles or 'heads'. The long head and lateral head combine to form the horseshoe shape at the top of your arm, while the medial head runs beneath the long head down to the elbow. Their job is to straighten your elbow, so they come into play every time you push something away from your body, such as when you do bench presses (see p94).

Because the arm muscles are relatively small, many people combine arm training with bigger muscle groups. Biceps training goes well with back training because they both involve pulling movements, while triceps and chest training go well together because they both involve pressing motions.

What follows is the best selection of exercises for building your biceps, triceps and forearms, plus variations so that you (and your muscles) don't get bored.

The key to effective arms training is to focus on the muscles you are working and don't allow larger muscle groups to take over by swinging your body.

Main exercises

Barbell curl	18
Seated dumb-bell curl	20
EZ-bar preacher curl	22
Hammer curl	24
Chin-up	26
Bench dip	28
Dip	30
Close-grip bench press	32
Lying triceps extension	34
Seated one-arm overhead triceps extension	36
Dumb-bell kickback	38
Triceps press down	40
Wrist curl	42

Barbell curl

Target: **biceps**

This is the classic biceps move, allowing you to move the maximum weight to develop mass in your biceps.

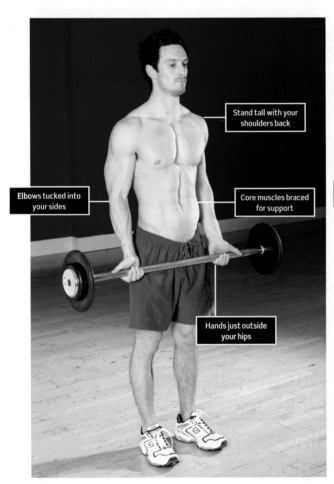

Stand tall with your shoulders back

Core muscles braced for support

Elbows tucked into your sides

Hands just outside your hips

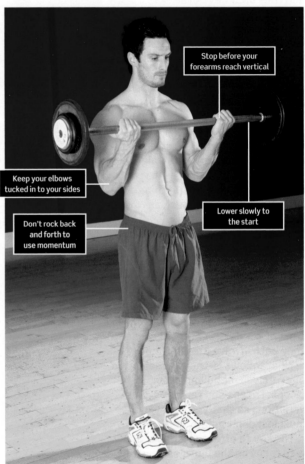

Stop before your forearms reach vertical

Keep your elbows tucked in to your sides

Lower slowly to the start

Don't rock back and forth to use momentum

Variations

EZ-BAR CURL

The EZ-bar allows you to turn your hands inwards slightly, taking some of the strain off your wrists and elbows.

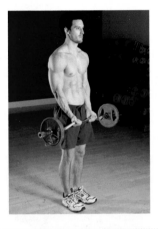
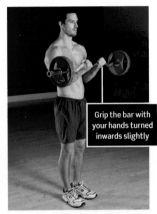

Grip the bar with your hands turned inwards slightly

DUMB-BELL CURL

With dumb-bells you work both arms evenly, unlike the barbell curl where your stronger arm can take more of the strain.

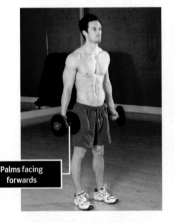
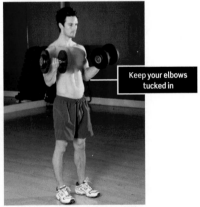

Palms facing forwards

Keep your elbows tucked in

NEGATIVE BARBELL CURL

Get a training partner to help you lift the bar into the 'up' position, then lower it as slowly as you can with good form. Focusing on the eccentric (lowering) phase allows you to use heavy weights and has great potential for muscle growth.

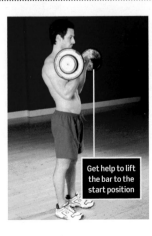
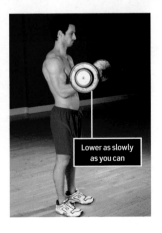

Get help to lift the bar to the start position

Lower as slowly as you can

Seated dumb-bell curl

Target: biceps

The seated position locks your hips into place so you can't uses momentum to start the move, placing all the emphasis on your biceps. Plus, by supinating (turning out) your wrists at the top of the move you place extra tension on your biceps brachii.

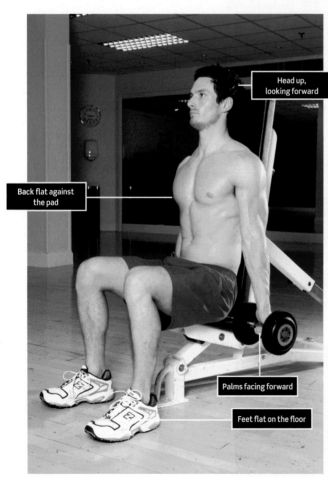

Head up, looking forward

Back flat against the pad

Palms facing forward

Feet flat on the floor

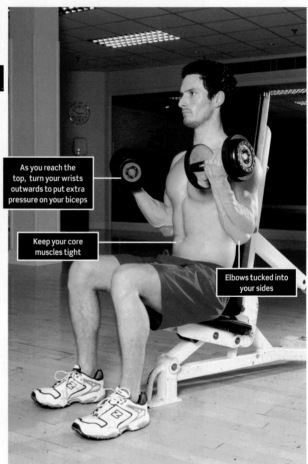

As you reach the top, turn your wrists outwards to put extra pressure on your biceps

Keep your core muscles tight

Elbows tucked into your sides

Variations

SWISS BALL DUMB-BELL CURL

Sitting on a Swiss ball requires you to hold your core muscles tight to prevent wobble, thus ensuring perfect posture for performing the dumb-bell curls.

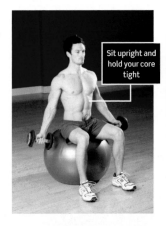
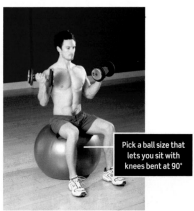

Sit upright and hold your core tight

Pick a ball size that lets you sit with knees bent at 90°

CONCENTRATION CURL

This move locks your elbow in place, preventing you from swinging your upper arm to help shift the weight. This means that all the stress is focused on the biceps, and you may need to use a lighter weight to perform the move correctly.

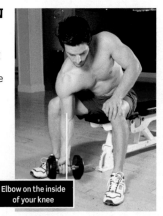
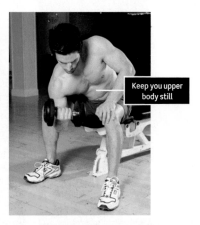

Elbow on the inside of your knee

Keep you upper body still

INCLINE DUMB-BELL CURL

By lying back on an incline bench, you maintain the resistance on your biceps throughout the full range of the curl. With seated curls the resistance can drop off towards the top of the move as your forearm gets near to vertical.

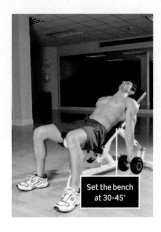
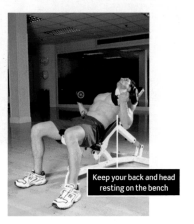

Set the bench at 30-45°

Keep your back and head resting on the bench

EZ-bar preacher curl

Target: biceps

The preacher bench stabilises your upper arms to fully isolate your biceps during curls. In this position, a barbell can place a lot of stress on your wrists, so an EZ-bar is a safer option.

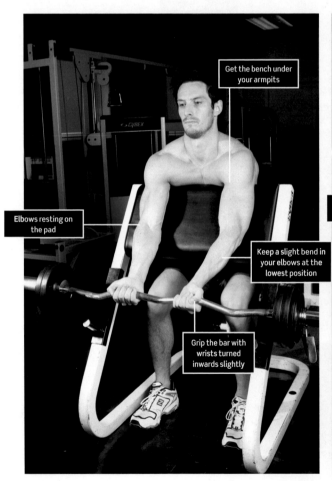

Get the bench under your armpits

Elbows resting on the pad

Keep a slight bend in your elbows at the lowest position

Grip the bar with wrists turned inwards slightly

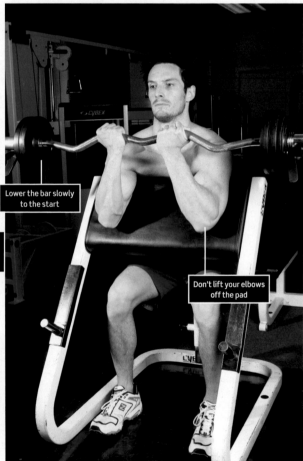

Lower the bar slowly to the start

Don't lift your elbows off the pad

Variations

SWISS BALL DUMB-BELL PREACHER CURL

The unstable platform requires you to concentrate on perfect form to prevent wobbling or collapsing on the floor. Use lighter weights to allow for this.

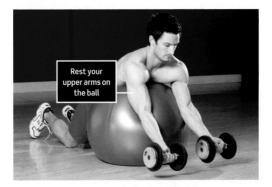

Rest your upper arms on the ball

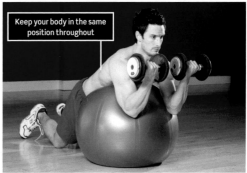

Keep your body in the same position throughout

ONE-ARM PREACHER CURL

Work each arm individually to ensure balanced growth in both biceps.

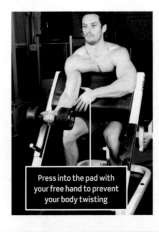

Press into the pad with your free hand to prevent your body twisting

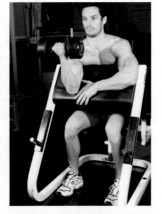

REVERSE EZ-BAR PREACHER CURL

Use an overhand grip to place the emphasis on the brachialis and brachioradialis muscles on your lower biceps and forearms.

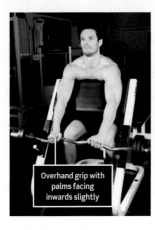

Overhand grip with palms facing inwards slightly

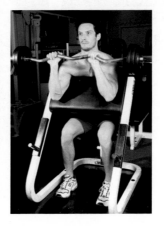

Hammer curl

Target: biceps

This neutral grip takes some of the emphasis away from your biceps brachii and places it on the brachioradialis muscles in your forearms.

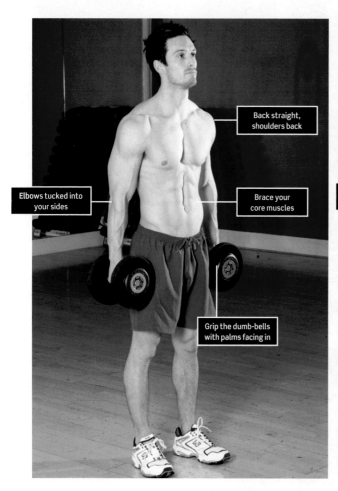

Back straight, shoulders back

Elbows tucked into your sides

Brace your core muscles

Grip the dumb-bells with palms facing in

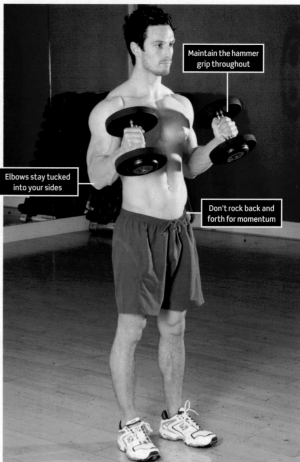

Maintain the hammer grip throughout

Elbows stay tucked into your sides

Don't rock back and forth for momentum

Variations

ROPE CABLE CURL

Using a cable ensures that the resistance remains the same at the top of the move as it does at the bottom.

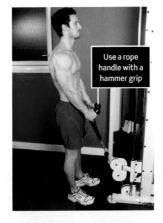
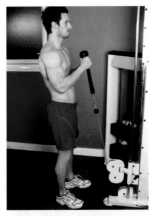

Use a rope handle with a hammer grip

ALTERNATING HAMMER CURL WITH TWIST

By curling one arm at a time you're less likely to lean back to initiate the move, and by supinating your wrists at the top of the move you hit your biceps from two angles at the same time.

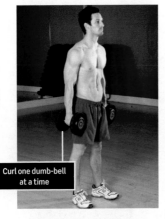
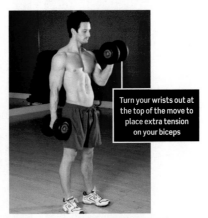

Curl one dumb-bell at a time

Turn your wrists out at the top of the move to place extra tension on your biceps

REVERSE CURL

Hold a barbell or dumb-bells with an overhand grip to transfer more of the emphasis to the brachialis.

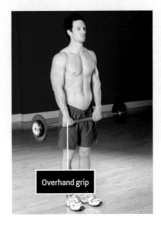
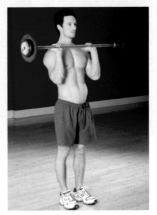

Overhand grip

Chin-up

Target: **biceps, lats (sides of back)**

Use an under-hand grip to make your biceps work hard, while your back muscles (among others) step in to aid this multi-joint move.

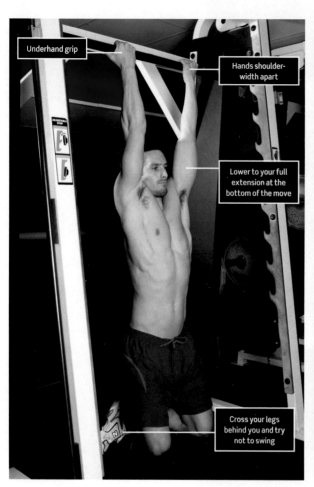

Underhand grip

Hands shoulder-width apart

Lower to your full extension at the bottom of the move

Cross your legs behind you and try not to swing

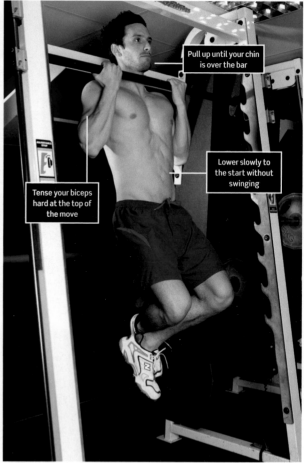

Pull up until your chin is over the bar

Lower slowly to the start without swinging

Tense your biceps hard at the top of the move

Variations

HAMMER GRIP CHIN-UP

Place greater emphasis on your brachialis and brachioradialis by using a neutral grip. If you don't have a pull-up machine with neutral handles, you can place a V-handle from a cable row machine over a pull-up bar to get the same effect.

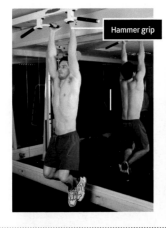

Hammer grip

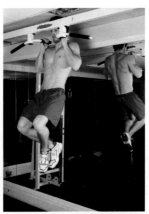

WEIGHTED CHIN-UP

If you find chin-ups easy, wear a weight belt to ensure that you reach failure within your chosen rep range.

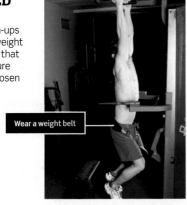

Wear a weight belt

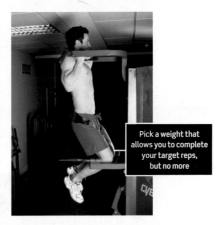

Pick a weight that allows you to complete your target reps, but no more

NEGATIVE CHIN-UP

If you find chin-ups difficult, use a bench or training partner to help you into the 'up' position and then lower yourself as slowly as you can. Repeat this exercise over several sessions until you can perform full chin-ups.

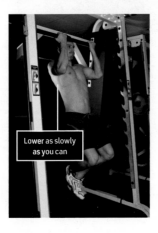

Lower as slowly as you can

Bench dip

Target: **triceps**

A compound bodyweight move that adds real mass to your triceps.

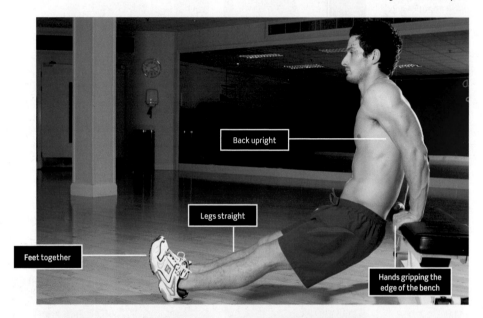

Back upright

Legs straight

Feet together

Hands gripping the edge of the bench

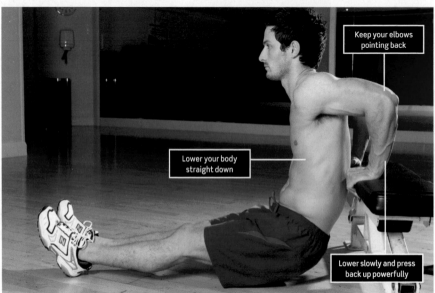

Keep your elbows pointing back

Lower your body straight down

Lower slowly and press back up powerfully

Variations

FEET UP BENCH DIP

Make the bench dip harder by raising your feet. This will also allow you a greater range of movement (if your elbow joints are up to it).

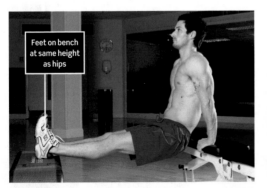

Feet on bench at same height as hips

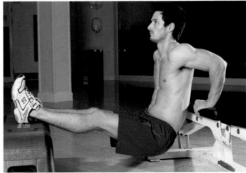

WEIGHTED BENCH DIP

If you find bench dips easy, adding weight will ensure you reach failure within your chosen rep range.

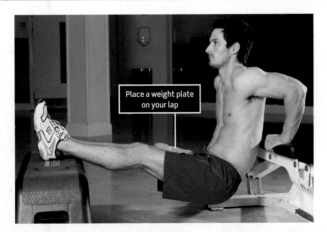

Place a weight plate on your lap

BENCH DIP WITH LEG LIFT

By lifting one leg as you dip, you introduce a rotational effect into the move, which forces your core muscles to work harder to maintain perfect form throughout.

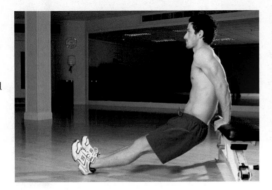

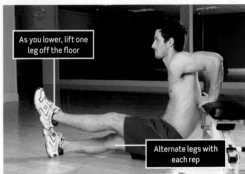

As you lower, lift one leg off the floor

Alternate legs with each rep

Dip

Target: **triceps, chest**

The big triceps move. This can be tough to get right at first, but keep at it if you want to add real power and mass to your upper arms.

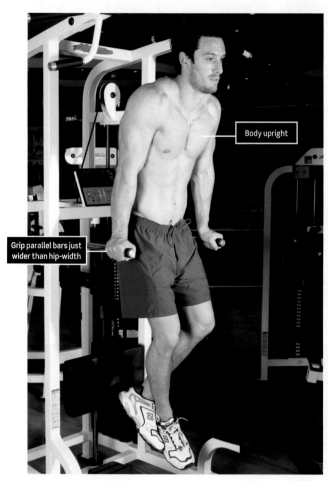

Body upright

Grip parallel bars just wider than hip-width

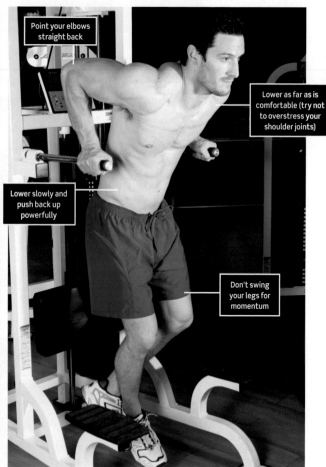

Point your elbows straight back

Lower as far as is comfortable (try not to overstress your shoulder joints)

Lower slowly and push back up powerfully

Don't swing your legs for momentum

Variations

ASSISTED DIP

If you struggle to do full dips, the dip machine can help you get started. A set of light dips is also a good way to warm up your delicate shoulder muscles before moving on to full dips.

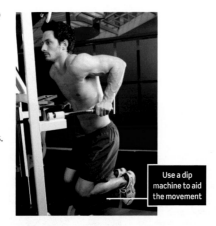

Use a dip machine to aid the movement

WEIGHTED DIP

If you find dips easy, hang a weight plate from your waist so that you hit failure within your chosen rep range.

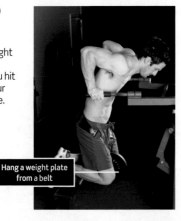

Hang a weight plate from a belt

FOLD DIP

By drawing in your knees and leaning forward during the dip, you can take some of the pressure off your shoulders because it lessens the angle between your torso and upper arms.

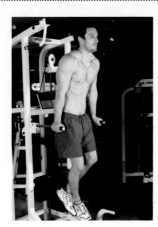

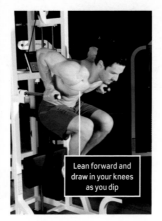

Lean forward and draw in your knees as you dip

Close-grip bench press

Target: triceps, chest

By bringing your hands close together for a bench press, you transfer much of the emphasis from your chest to your triceps.

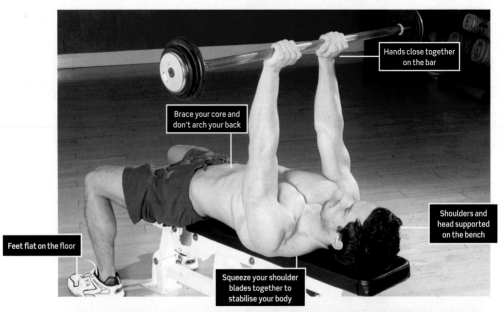

Hands close together on the bar

Brace your core and don't arch your back

Shoulders and head supported on the bench

Feet flat on the floor

Squeeze your shoulder blades together to stabilise your body

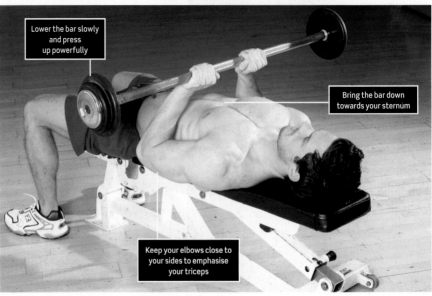

Lower the bar slowly and press up powerfully

Bring the bar down towards your sternum

Keep your elbows close to your sides to emphasise your triceps

Variations

DIAMOND PRESS-UP

Touch your thumbs and index fingers together (they make the shape of a diamond) to focus the workload on your triceps while doing press-ups.

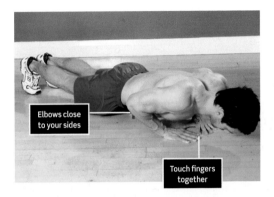

Elbows close to your sides

Touch fingers together

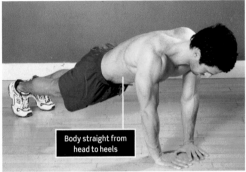

Body straight from head to heels

UNILATERAL WALL PRESS-UP

You need to keep your elbow tucked in to maintain balance, which places the emphasis on your triceps. To make the move harder stand further away from the wall.

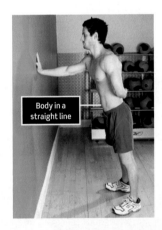

Body in a straight line

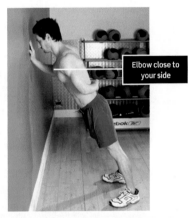

Elbow close to your side

MEDICINE BALL CLOSE-GRIP PRESS-UP

The medicine ball adds wobble to a diamond press-up, forcing the stabilising muscles in your core and shoulders to work harder.

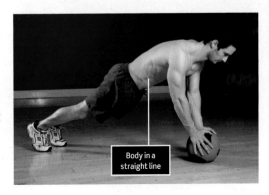

Body in a straight line

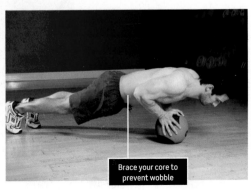

Brace your core to prevent wobble

Lying triceps extension

Target: **triceps**
Blast your triceps' long head with
this focused EZ-bar movement.

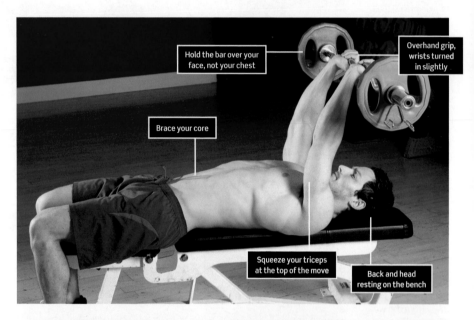

Hold the bar over your
face, not your chest

Overhand grip,
wrists turned
in slightly

Brace your core

Squeeze your triceps
at the top of the move

Back and head
resting on the bench

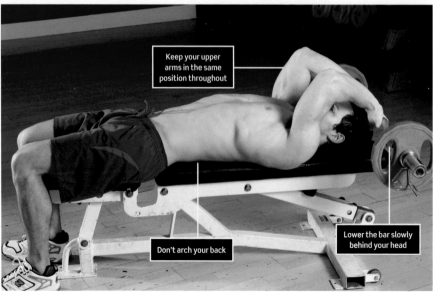

Keep your upper
arms in the same
position throughout

Don't arch your back

Lower the bar slowly
behind your head

Variations

REVERSE GRIP LYING TRICEPS EXTENSION

By holding the bar with an underhand grip you shift the emphasis to the triceps' lateral head.

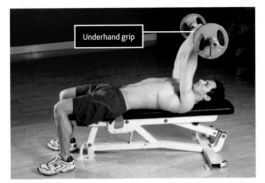

Underhand grip

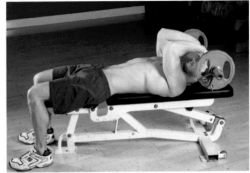

DUMB-BELL LYING TRICEPS EXTENSION

Work both triceps in isolation by using dumb-bells. This also helps if you have weaknesses in your shoulder girdle that can be exacerbated by using a bar that locks your wrists into place.

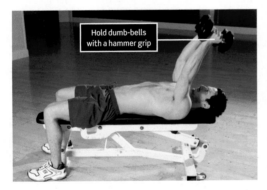

Hold dumb-bells with a hammer grip

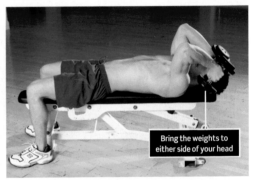

Bring the weights to either side of your head

SWISS BALL LYING TRICEPS EXTENSION

Add extra wobble to give your core a thorough workout at the same time.

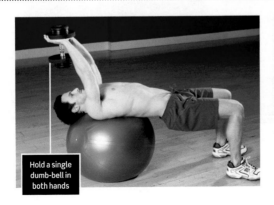

Hold a single dumb-bell in both hands

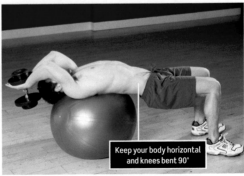

Keep your body horizontal and knees bent 90°

Seated one-arm overhead triceps extension

Target: triceps

Add shape and definition to your triceps by targeting each arm separately.

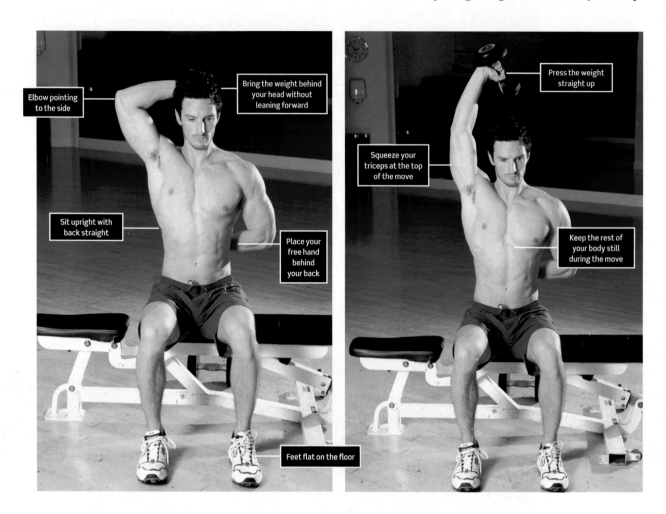

Elbow pointing to the side

Bring the weight behind your head without leaning forward

Press the weight straight up

Sit upright with back straight

Squeeze your triceps at the top of the move

Place your free hand behind your back

Keep the rest of your body still during the move

Feet flat on the floor

Variations

SWISS BALL ONE-ARM OVERHEAD TRICEPS EXTENSION

The Swiss ball forces you to maintain good posture throughout the move, and to perform the move with perfect form.

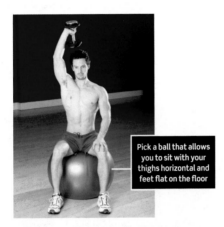

Pick a ball that allows you to sit with your thighs horizontal and feet flat on the floor

SEATED EZ-BAR OVERHEAD TRICEPS EXTENSION

Using an EZ-bar allows you to press more weight, meaning bigger muscle gains.

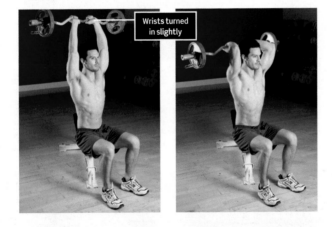

Wrists turned in slightly

DUMB-BELL OVERHEAD TRICEPS EXTENSION

If you don't have an EZ-bar you can place both hands on a dumb-bell. Some people will find this places less of a twisting force at the elbows and shoulders than can happen with an EZ-bar.

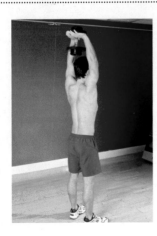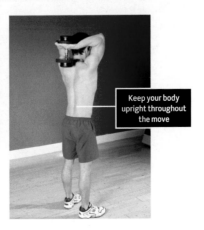

Keep your body upright throughout the move

Dumb-bell kickback

Target: **triceps**

This move hits your triceps from a new angle, placing additional force on the muscle at the top of the move compared to the overhead triceps extension.

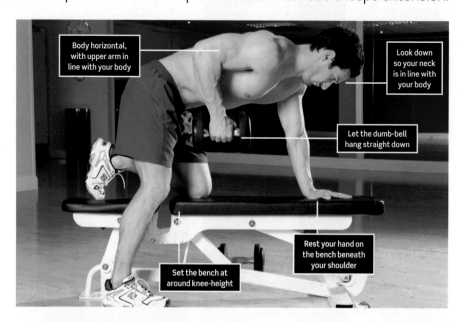

Body horizontal, with upper arm in line with your body

Look down so your neck is in line with your body

Let the dumb-bell hang straight down

Rest your hand on the bench beneath your shoulder

Set the bench at around knee-height

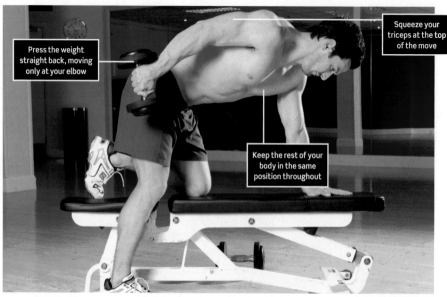

Squeeze your triceps at the **top** of the move

Press the weight straight back, moving only at your elbow

Keep the rest of your body in the same position throughout

Variations

DUMB-BELL KICKBACK WITH LIFT

After performing a dumb-bell kickback, lift your straight arm above the horizontal to place greater emphasis on the long head of your triceps.

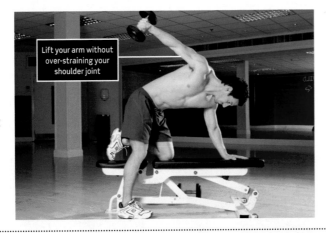

Lift your arm without over-straining your shoulder joint

TWO-ARM KICKBACK

Work both arms at the same time – but you need to be strong in the core to maintain this position.

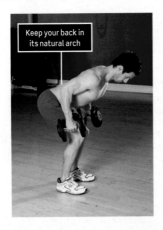

Keep your back in its natural arch

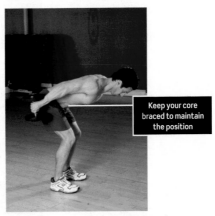

Keep your core braced to maintain the position

CABLE KICKBACK

The cable places greater force on your muscles at the beginning of the move compared to the dumb-bell kickback.

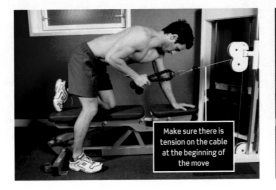

Make sure there is tension on the cable at the beginning of the move

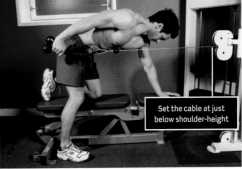

Set the cable at just below shoulder-height

Triceps press down

Target: **triceps**

This exercise is easy to perform and the cable provides resistance across the full range of the move.

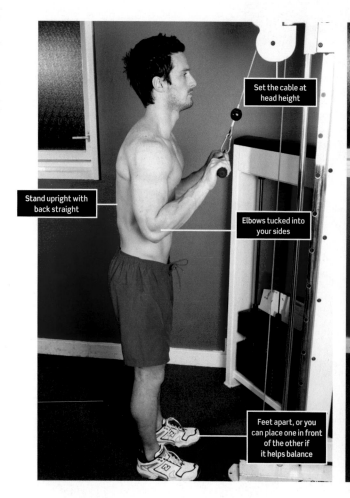

Set the cable at head height

Stand upright with back straight

Elbows tucked into your sides

Feet apart, or you can place one in front of the other if it helps balance

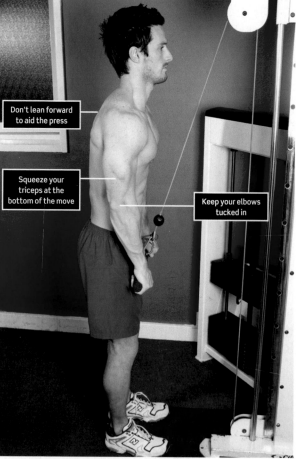

Don't lean forward to aid the press

Squeeze your triceps at the bottom of the move

Keep your elbows tucked in

Variations

ROPE PRESS DOWN
Using a rope gives you an intense contraction at the bottom of the move.

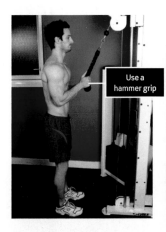

Use a hammer grip

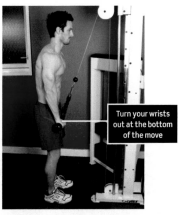

Turn your wrists out at the bottom of the move

REVERSE GRIP PRESS DOWN
By swapping to an underhand grip you shift the emphasis to the triceps' lateral head.

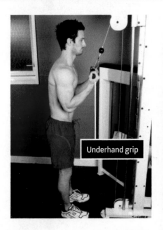

Underhand grip

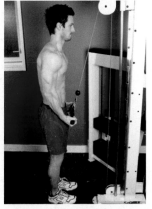

UNILATERAL PRESS DOWN
Get balanced gains by working each arm individually.

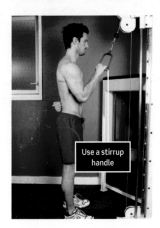

Use a stirrup handle

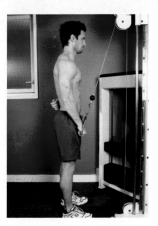

Wrist curl

Target: forearms

Build your forearms and get a crushing grip.

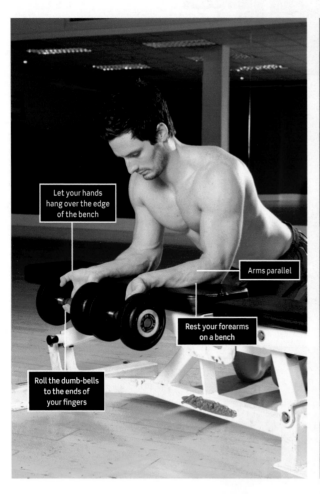

Let your hands hang over the edge of the bench

Arms parallel

Rest your forearms on a bench

Roll the dumb-bells to the ends of your fingers

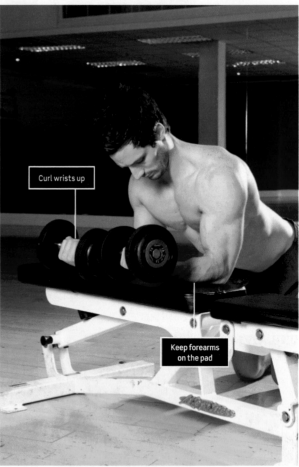

Curl wrists up

Keep forearms on the pad

Variations

REVERSE WRIST CURL

Hit your forearms from the opposite side.

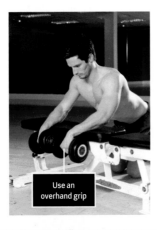

Use an overhand grip

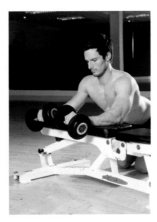

FOREARM ROTATION

Add a rotational aspect to your forearm workout, which will add strength to your smashes in racquet sports.

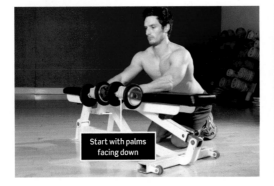

Start with palms facing down

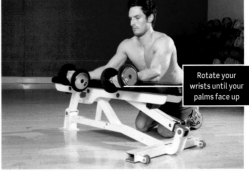

Rotate your wrists until your palms face up

BARBELL COLLAR GRIP

Get a powerful handshake using the barbell collars, or crush a rubber ball for the same effect.

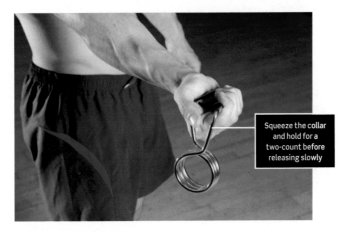

Squeeze the collar and hold for a two-count before releasing slowly

ABS

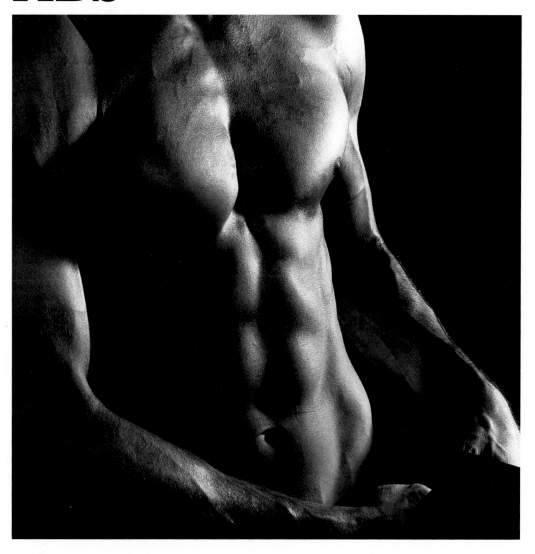

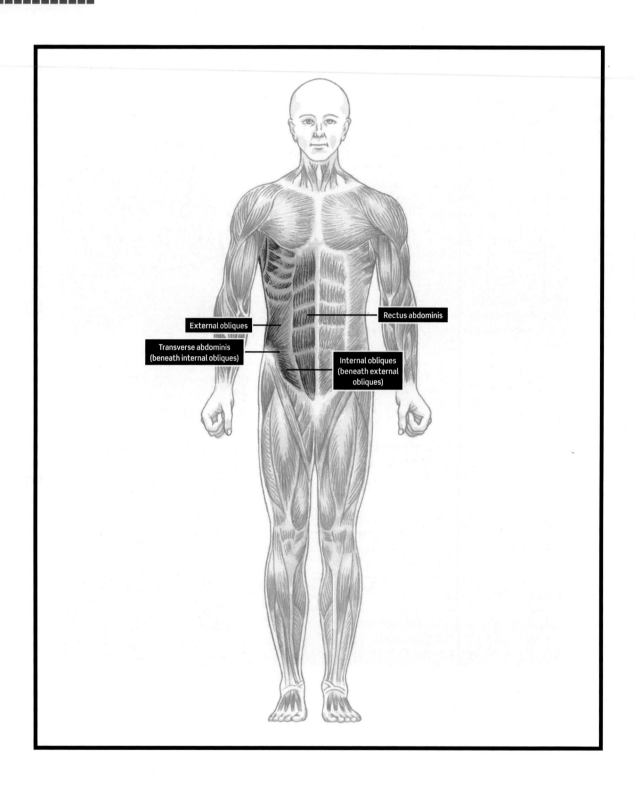

External obliques

Rectus abdominis

Transverse abdominis
(beneath internal obliques)

Internal obliques
(beneath external
obliques)

ABS

Washboard abs are high on every man's list of must-have muscles, yet they often cause confusion when it comes to training.

The first mistake that many men make is to think that more is always better. They crank out hundreds of crunches a day and wonder why those little squares of muscle aren't developing properly. The reason is that, like any other muscle, the way to build your abdominals is to keep the reps per set fairly low – in the region of 10-12 – and increase the resistance when you find it too easy, not the number of reps. That means adding weight when doing crunches or using a cable machine.

The other mistake that men often make when hunting for abs is to forget about the layer of fat that covers them. Men tend store fat around the gut, so you really need to work hard at lowering your overall body fat percentage if you want to see your abs. This means watching your diet (see p182) and doing plenty of big muscle moves, such as squats and deadlifts, that torch calories.

Your six-pack is actually one sheet of muscle, called the rectus abdominis, which extends from your ribcage to your pubic bone. Because it is one muscle, any abs-specific exercise will work the entire area, but it is possible to target the upper or lower portions of the rectus abdominis with different exercises, which is why we have indicated on the exercises whether a move focuses on the upper or lower abs.

Your rectus abdominis is supported on either side by your external obliques and by the internal obliques and transverse abdominis that lie beneath the external obliques. Together they support and manipulate your spine, and combine with your lower-back muscles to form your 'core' – the muscular region that connects your upper and lower body. A strong core is vital for performing any dynamic movements in sport and for preventing back pain. So abs training is not just for show: it will make you stand taller and perform better in all areas of life.

Main exercises

Crunch	48
Reverse crunch	50
Oblique crunch	52
Crossover crunch	54
Knee raise	56
Plank	58
Side plank	60
Bench leg raise	62
Jacknife	64
Seated Russian twist	66
Barbell rollout	68

Crunch

Target: **upper abdominals**

The classic move for targeting your upper abs – and still one of the best.

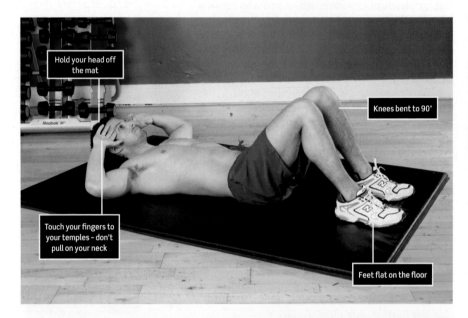

Hold your head off the mat

Knees bent to 90°

Touch your fingers to your temples – don't pull on your neck

Feet flat on the floor

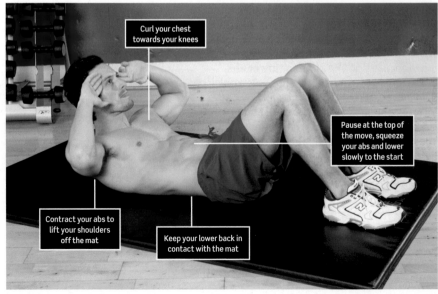

Curl your chest towards your knees

Pause at the top of the move, squeeze your abs and lower slowly to the start

Contract your abs to lift your shoulders off the mat

Keep your lower back in contact with the mat

Variations

SWISS BALL CRUNCH

Lying on a Swiss ball works your core harder to stabilise your body and allows for a greater range of movement when doing the crunch.

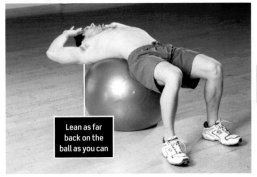

Lean as far back on the ball as you can

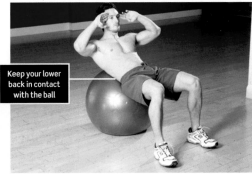

Keep your lower back in contact with the ball

WEIGHTED CRUNCH

If crunches are easy for you, rather than doing more reps, try adding weight to increase the intensity of the move and stimulate more muscle growth.

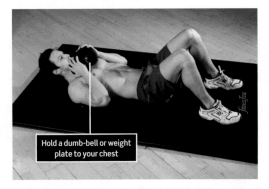

Hold a dumb-bell or weight plate to your chest

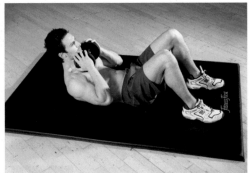

CABLE CRUNCH

The cable requires you to crunch against a constant force

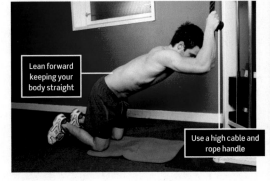

Lean forward keeping your body straight

Use a high cable and rope handle

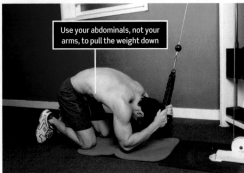

Use your abdominals, not your arms, to pull the weight down

Reverse crunch

Target: **lower abdominals**

Place the emphasis on the lower part of your abs by attacking them from a different angle.

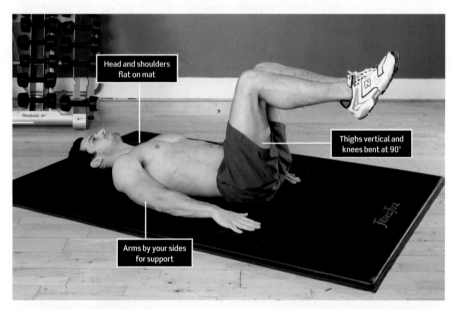

Head and shoulders flat on mat

Thighs vertical and knees bent at 90°

Arms by your sides for support

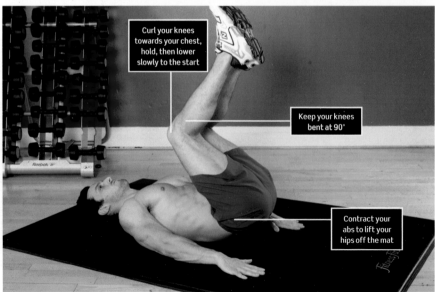

Curl your knees towards your chest, hold, then lower slowly to the start

Keep your knees bent at 90°

Contract your abs to lift your hips off the mat

Variations

MEDICINE BALL REVERSE CRUNCH

The extra weight will stimulate extra muscle growth. And using a medicine ball safeguards you from dropping a dumb-bell on your head.

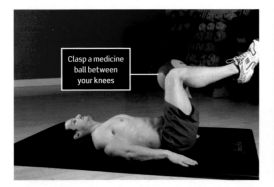

Clasp a medicine ball between your knees

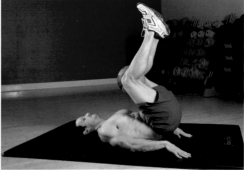

TUCK AND CRUNCH

Attack your abs from above and below at the same time.

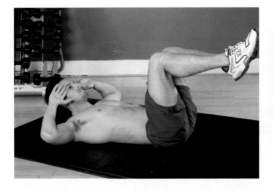

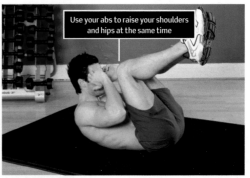

Use your abs to raise your shoulders and hips at the same time

SEATED REVERSE CRUNCH

By sitting on the edge of a bench you increase the workload on your lower abs and force your core to work harder to balance your body.

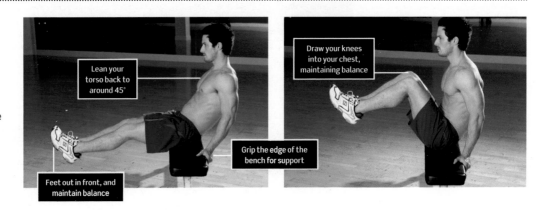

Lean your torso back to around 45°

Grip the edge of the bench for support

Feet out in front, and maintain balance

Draw your knees into your chest, maintaining balance

Oblique crunch

Target: obliques (side abs)

Hit your abs from the side to target the obliques, the muscles that frame your six-pack.

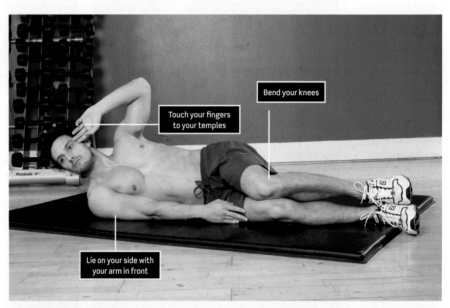

Touch your fingers to your temples

Bend your knees

Lie on your side with your arm in front

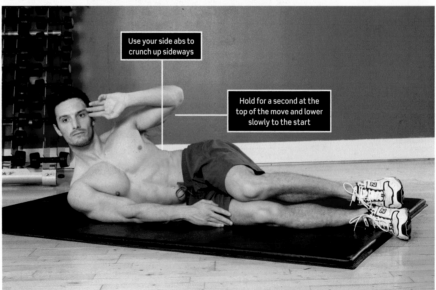

Use your side abs to crunch up sideways

Hold for a second at the top of the move and lower slowly to the start

Variations

SWISS BALL OBLIQUE CRUNCH

Get a greater range of movement by wrapping your body around the ball.

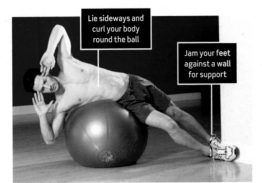

Lie sideways and curl your body round the ball

Jam your feet against a wall for support

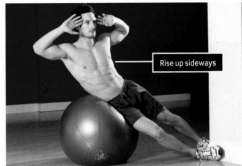

Rise up sideways

DUMB-BELL SIDE BEND

Vary the resistance you place on your obliques by using a dumb-bell.

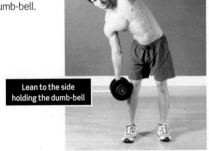

Lean to the side holding the dumb-bell

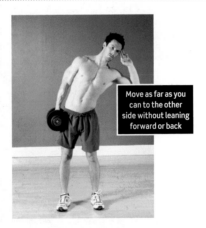

Move as far as you can to the other side without leaning forward or back

MEDICINE BALL SIDE THROWDOWNS

This dynamic throwing movement adds a plyometric element to your workout, which fires up your fast-twitch muscle fibres.

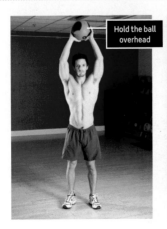

Hold the ball overhead

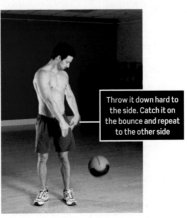

Throw it down hard to the side. Catch it on the bounce and repeat to the other side

Crossover crunch

Target: **abdominals**

Add a twist to your crunch to hit your abs from several angles at once.

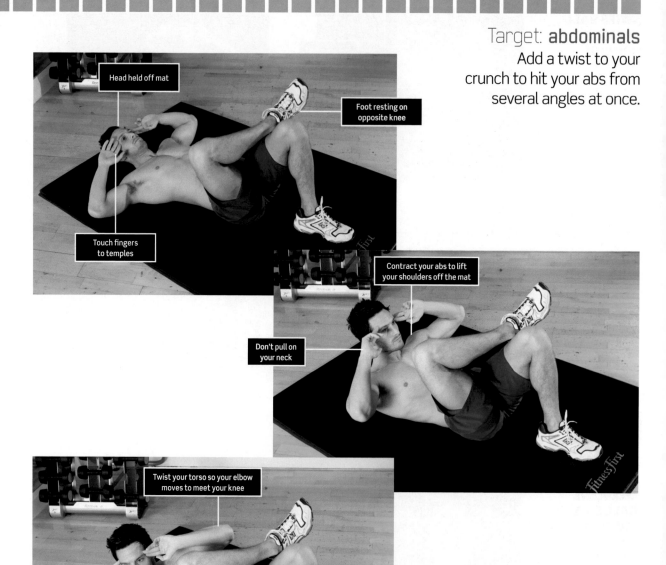

Head held off mat

Foot resting on opposite knee

Touch fingers to temples

Contract your abs to lift your shoulders off the mat

Don't pull on your neck

Twist your torso so your elbow moves to meet your knee

Reverse the move slowly back to the start

Variations

SWISS BALL TWIST CRUNCH

Get more range on the move and work your stabiliser muscles into the bargain.

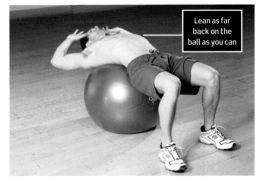

Lean as far back on the ball as you can

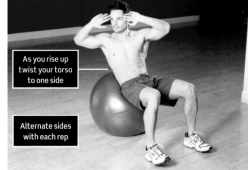

As you rise up twist your torso to one side

Alternate sides with each rep

BICYCLES

Do this move quickly to fully exhaust your abdominals.

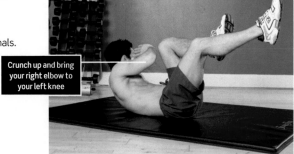

Crunch up and bring your right elbow to your left knee

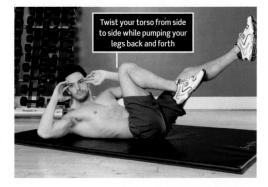

Twist your torso from side to side while pumping your legs back and forth

ONE-ARM CABLE CROSS CRUNCH

Crunch and twist against resistance to give your six-pack a thorough workout.

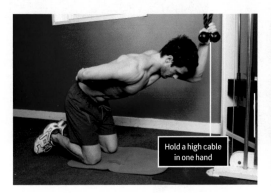

Hold a high cable in one hand

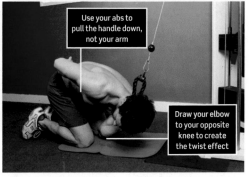

Use your abs to pull the handle down, not your arm

Draw your elbow to your opposite knee to create the twist effect

Knee raise

Target: **lower abdominals**

A tough move that really works your lower abs. If you're feeling strong you can hang from a pull-up bar, or you can rest on dip bars or use elbow straps to take your weight.

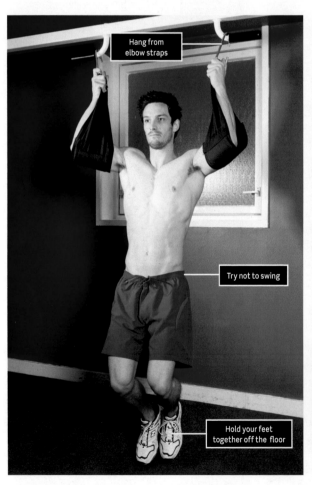

Hang from elbow straps

Try not to swing

Hold your feet together off the floor

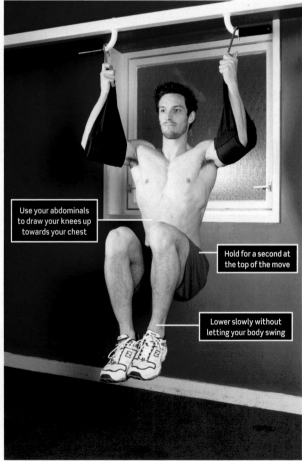

Use your abdominals to draw your knees up towards your chest

Hold for a second at the top of the move

Lower slowly without letting your body swing

Variations

LEG RAISE

Make the move tougher by straightening your legs.

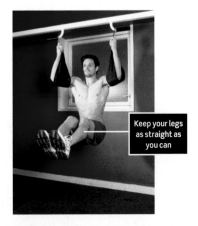

Keep your legs as straight as you can

TWISTING KNEE RAISE

Bring your obliques into play by raising and twisting your knees at the same time.

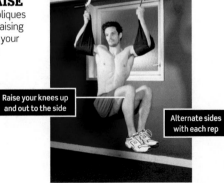

Raise your knees up and out to the side

Alternate sides with each rep

MEDICINE BALL KNEE RAISE

When you get good at knee raises you can add resistance so that you continue to reach failure within your chosen rep range.

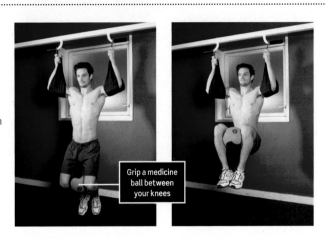

Grip a medicine ball between your knees

Plank

Target: core

Build a strong link between your upper and lower body with this classic stability move.

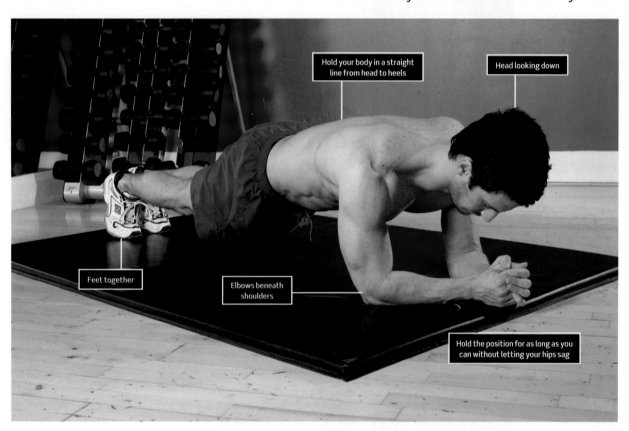

Hold your body in a straight line from head to heels

Head looking down

Feet together

Elbows beneath shoulders

Hold the position for as long as you can without letting your hips sag

Variations

SWISS BALL PLANK

The extra wobble forces your core stabilising muscles to work even harder.

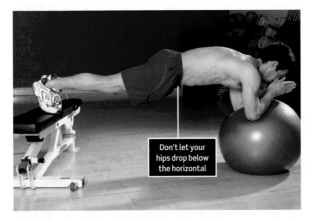

Don't let your hips drop below the horizontal

ONE-ARM ONE LEG PLANK

By lifting opposing arms and legs you introduce a rotational force that makes your midsection work harder to keep your body straight.

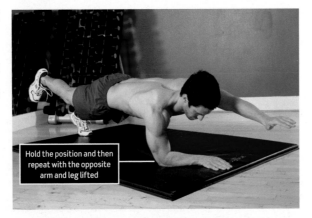

Hold the position and then repeat with the opposite arm and leg lifted

FOOT RAISE AND HOLD

This isometric hold targets your lower abs and will help you to maintain a strong core during heavy lifts.

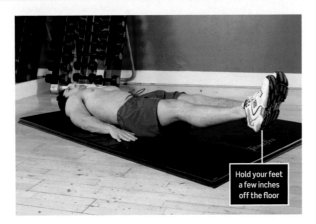

Hold your feet a few inches off the floor

Side plank

Target: core

Hold your body straight to build a powerful core
that will improve posture and sports performance.

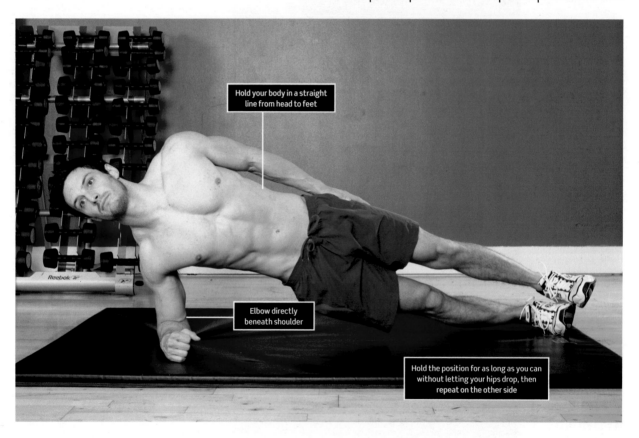

Hold your body in a straight
line from head to feet

Elbow directly
beneath shoulder

Hold the position for as long as you can
without letting your hips drop, then
repeat on the other side

Variations

SWISS BALL SIDE PLANK

The extra instability makes holding the position tougher.

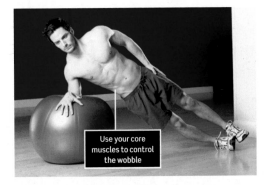

Use your core muscles to control the wobble

RAISED SIDE PLANK

Lifting and arm and a leg introduces other muscles into the hold and makes your core work harder to maintain balance.

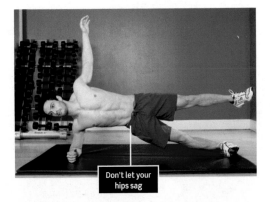

Don't let your hips sag

SIDE PLANK WITH LATERAL RAISE

Use a light dumb-bell – this move is more about improving co-ordination than building muscle.

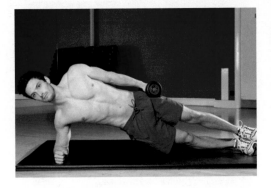
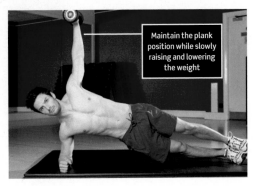

Maintain the plank position while slowly raising and lowering the weight

Bench leg raise

Target: abdominals, hip flexors

This move targets both the abs and the muscles at the front of your groin, which work together when you raise your legs, such as when you kick a ball.

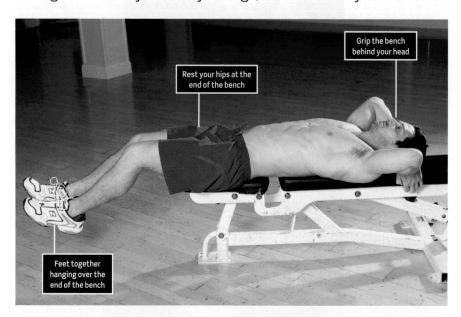

Grip the bench behind your head

Rest your hips at the end of the bench

Feet together hanging over the end of the bench

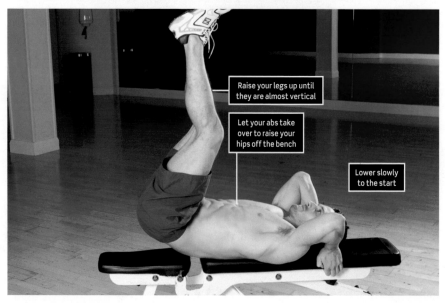

Raise your legs up until they are almost vertical

Let your abs take over to raise your hips off the bench

Lower slowly to the start

Variations

HIP RAISE

Lift your bum off the floor to place extra work on your abs and hips.

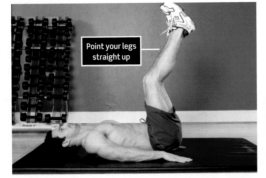

Point your legs straight up

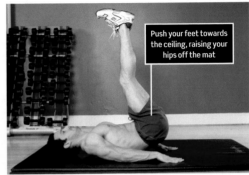

Push your feet towards the ceiling, raising your hips off the mat

WEIGHTED HIP RAISE

Hold a dumb-bell in your feet to increase the resistance – just don't drop it on your head!

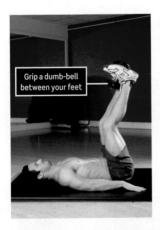

Grip a dumb-bell between your feet

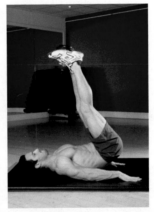

MEDICINE BALL LEG DROP

Make your abs, hips and adductors (the insides of your thighs) work hard with this medicine ball move.

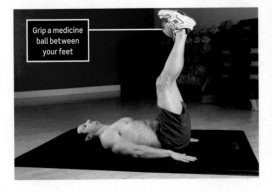

Grip a medicine ball between your feet

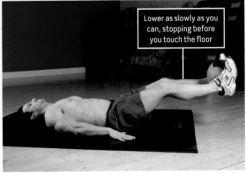

Lower as slowly as you can, stopping before you touch the floor

Jacknife

Target: **upper and lower abdominals**

Make your abs sing with this advanced move that requires flexibility as well as a strong core.

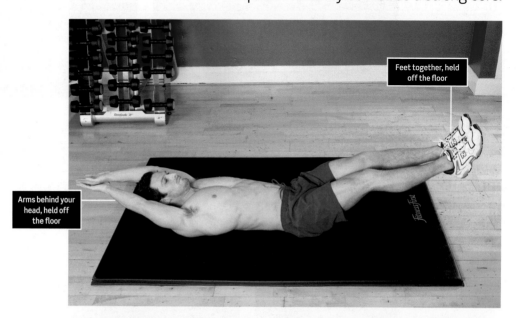

Feet together, held off the floor

Arms behind your head, held off the floor

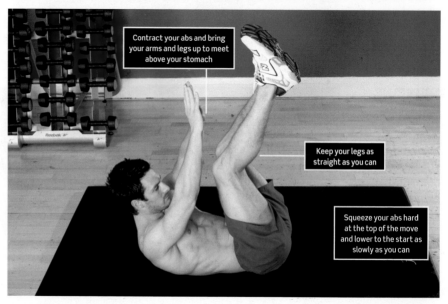

Contract your abs and bring your arms and legs up to meet above your stomach

Keep your legs as straight as you can

Squeeze your abs hard at the top of the move and lower to the start as slowly as you can

Variations

SWISS BALL JACKNIFE

This moves takes gravity out of the equation but adds in extra wobble to keep your core stabiliser muscles working hard.

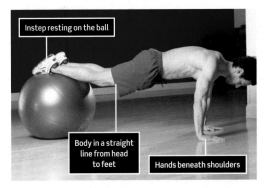

Instep resting on the ball

Body in a straight line from head to feet

Hands beneath shoulders

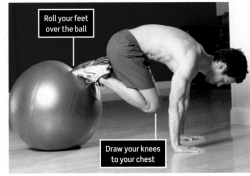

Roll your feet over the ball

Draw your knees to your chest

MODIFIED V-SIT

If the jacknife proves too hard, this move targets the same muscles without placing so much strain on your hamstrings and lower back.

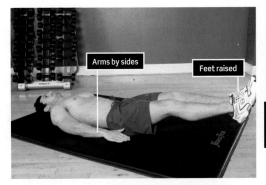

Arms by sides

Feet raised

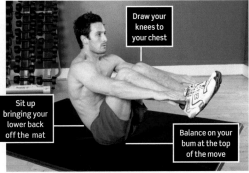

Draw your knees to your chest

Sit up bringing your lower back off the mat

Balance on your bum at the top of the move

SWISS BALL PASSING JACKNIFE

Pass the ball from hands to feet to ensure that you maintain perfect form at all times.

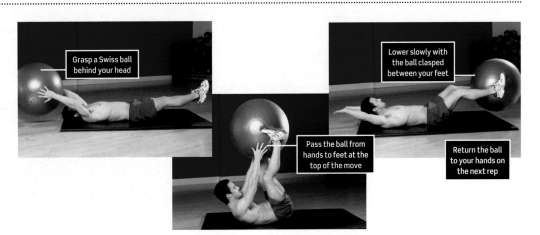

Grasp a Swiss ball behind your head

Lower slowly with the ball clasped between your feet

Pass the ball from hands to feet at the top of the move

Return the ball to your hands on the next rep

Seated Russian twist

This rotational move works your obliques and entire core to give you a strong foundation for all sports.

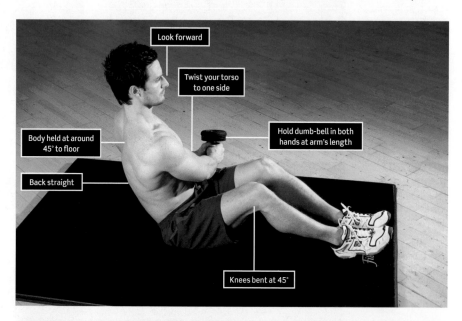

Look forward

Twist your torso to one side

Hold dumb-bell in both hands at arm's length

Body held at around 45° to floor

Back straight

Knees bent at 45°

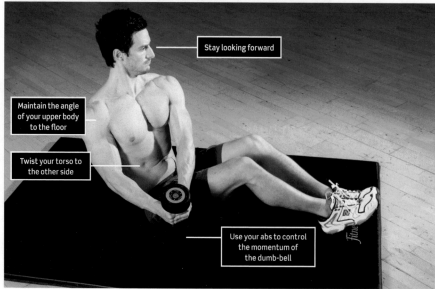

Stay looking forward

Maintain the angle of your upper body to the floor

Twist your torso to the other side

Use your abs to control the momentum of the dumb-bell

Variations

SWISS BALL RUSSIAN TWIST

The Swiss ball makes this move easier on your lower back but still makes your core work hard to stabilise the wobble.

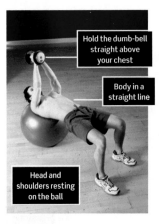

Hold the dumb-bell straight above your chest

Body in a straight line

Head and shoulders resting on the ball

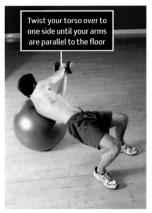

Twist your torso over to one side until your arms are parallel to the floor

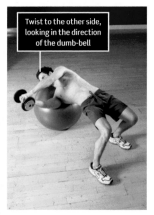

Twist to the other side, looking in the direction of the dumb-bell

LOWER-BODY RUSSIAN TWIST

Transfer the rotational emphasis to the lower part of your abdominals.

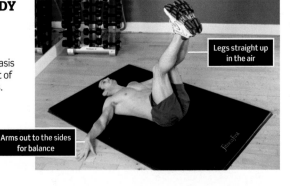

Legs straight up in the air

Arms out to the sides for balance

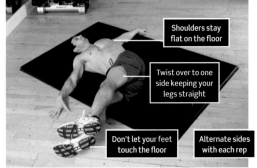

Shoulders stay flat on the floor

Twist over to one side keeping your legs straight

Don't let your feet touch the floor

Alternate sides with each rep

STANDING CABLE RUSSIAN TWIST

The cable provides a constant resistance as you turn your torso.

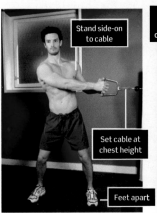

Stand side-on to cable

Set cable at chest height

Feet apart

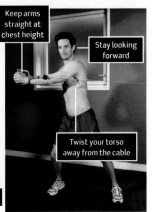

Keep arms straight at chest height

Stay looking forward

Twist your torso away from the cable

Barbell rollout

Target: core

Make your abs and lower back work together to stabilise your body in this move, which you can make as easy or as hard as you like.

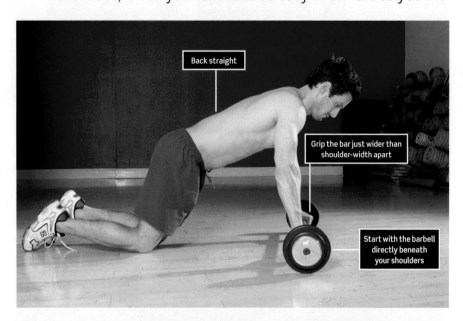

Back straight

Grip the bar just wider than shoulder-width apart

Start with the barbell directly beneath your shoulders

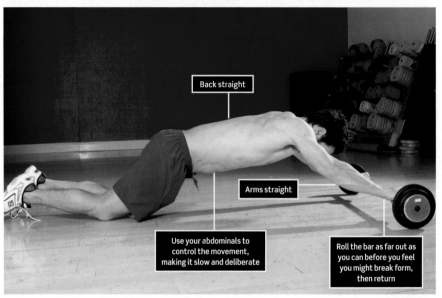

Back straight

Arms straight

Use your abdominals to control the movement, making it slow and deliberate

Roll the bar as far out as you can before you feel you might break form, then return

Variations

SWISS BALL ROLLOUT

This variation places less strain on your lower back but makes your core work hard to stabilise the wobble.

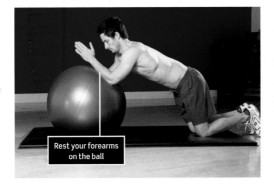

Rest your forearms on the ball

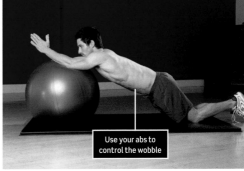

Use your abs to control the wobble

TOWEL SLIDE FLYE

This brings your chest and shoulders into play for a really testing upper-body move.

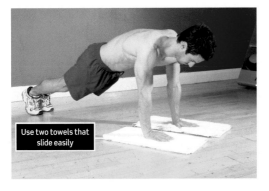

Use two towels that slide easily

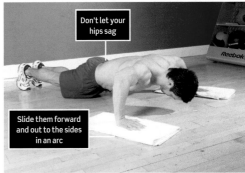

Don't let your hips sag

Slide them forward and out to the sides in an arc

SQUAT THRUSTS

Jump your feet back and forth to really work your core muscles and get your heart racing into the bargain.

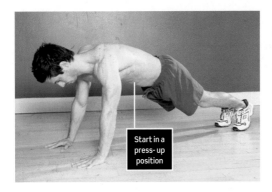

Start in a press-up position

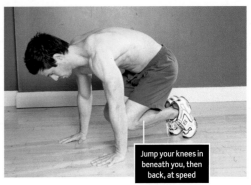

Jump your knees in beneath you, then back, at speed

BACK

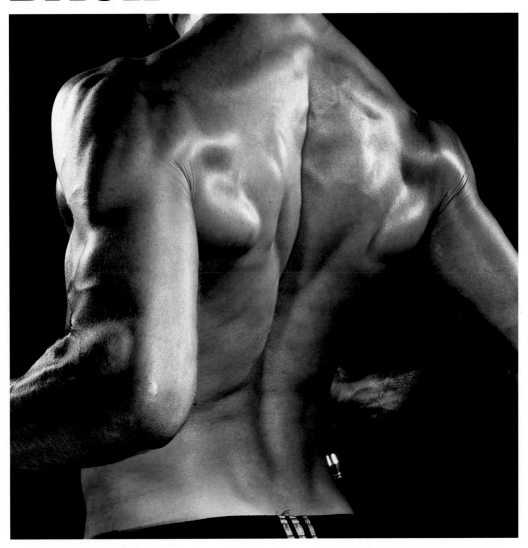

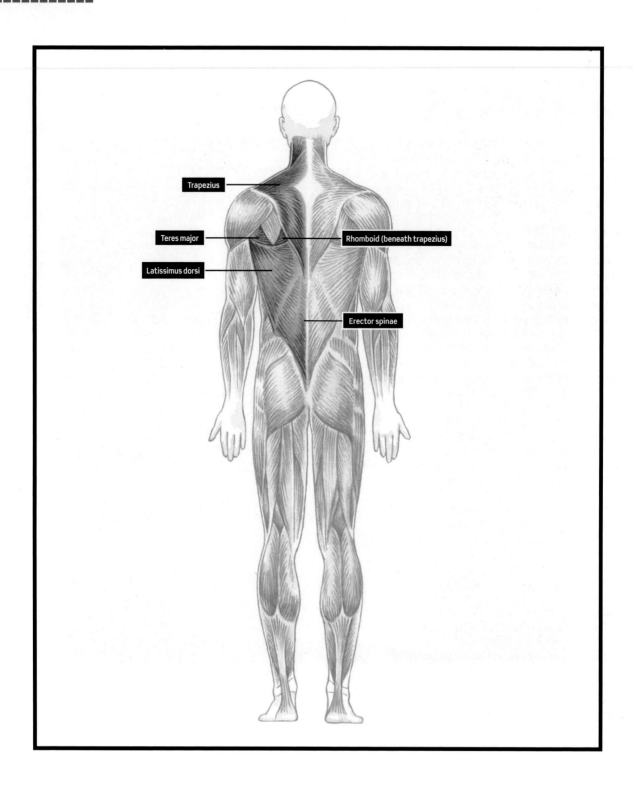

Trapezius

Teres major

Latissimus dorsi

Rhomboid (beneath trapezius)

Erector spinae

BACK

The poor old back muscles never get a look-in, literally. When you view your body in the mirror you can't see your back, so it's tempting to ignore your back muscles during training and concentrate on the glory muscles at the front – chest, abs and biceps. However, you ignore your back at your peril.

Not only does a strong back improve your physique, it helps to correct your posture and prevent injury. If, like many men, you spend hours in the gym doing bench presses but give little attention to your back, the over-developed muscles in your chest and front shoulders will pull your shoulders forward, making you look hunched like a gorilla, which is fine if that's the look you're aiming for, but not so good if you prefer to look like a Homo sapien. Also, a muscle imbalance from too little back training can lead to a lack of flexibility at the shoulder, which can in turn lead to injuries from badly performed exercises. The moral is: pay as much attention to your back as your front.

Your upper back is criss-crossed with muscles that manipulate your shoulders, allowing you to pull objects towards you and make a shrugging motion. The trapezius (traps) originate at your neck and spread out across your shoulder blades and down your spine. Beneath your arms, your latissimus dorsi (lats) are the wide wings that draw your arms down and in, such as when you do pull-ups. These large muscles are supported by a host of smaller ones that allow your arms and spine to move in a multitude of planes.

Running down the sides of your back bone, the erector spinae muscles do the job of supporting and stabilising your spine whenever you bend. These are the muscles that, if trained properly, will protect you from lower back pain when you do heavy lifts. Along with your abdominal muscles, the erector spinae form part of the 'core' that we refer to on many occasions in this book.

Main exercises

Bent-over row	74
Cable row	76
One-arm row	78
Pull-up	80
Lat pull-down	82
Shrug	84
Good morning	86
Two-point box	88

Bent-over row

Target: **traps, lats, rhomboids**
One of the original big-muscle moves.

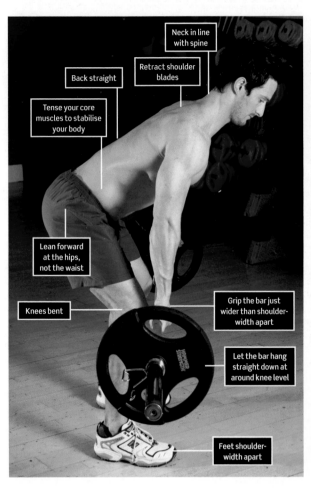

Neck in line
with spine

Retract shoulder
blades

Back straight

Tense your core
muscles to stabilise
your body

Lean forward
at the hips,
not the waist

Knees bent

Grip the bar just
wider than shoulder-
width apart

Let the bar hang
straight down at
around knee level

Feet shoulder-
width apart

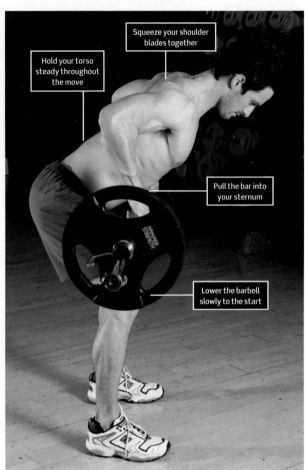

Squeeze your shoulder
blades together

Hold your torso
steady throughout
the move

Pull the bar into
your sternum

Lower the barbell
slowly to the start

Variations

DUMB-BELL BENT-OVER ROW

Requires a bit more co-ordination than the barbell version and prevents the stronger side of your body doing all the work.

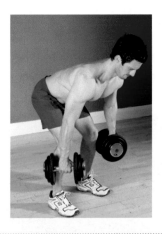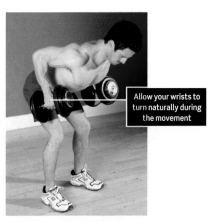

Allow your wrists to turn naturally during the movement

REVERSE GRIP BENT-OVER ROW

By reversing the grip you target your lats and lower traps more.

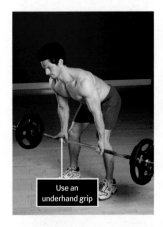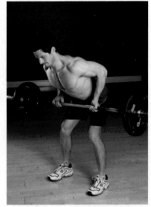

Use an underhand grip

BENT-OVER FLYE

This move uses lighter weights but allows you to get a really strong scapular retraction (the action of pulling your shoulder blades together).

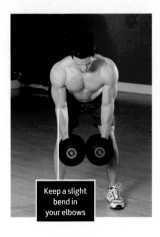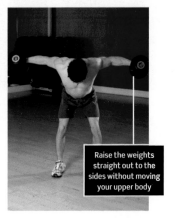

Keep a slight bend in your elbows

Raise the weights straight out to the sides without moving your upper body

Cable row

Target: **mid traps, lats, rhomboid**

Ensure perfect form for this move and it will repay you with real muscle-mass gains.

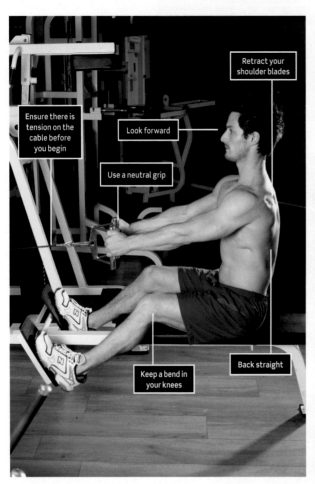

Retract your shoulder blades

Ensure there is tension on the cable before you begin

Look forward

Use a neutral grip

Keep a bend in your knees

Back straight

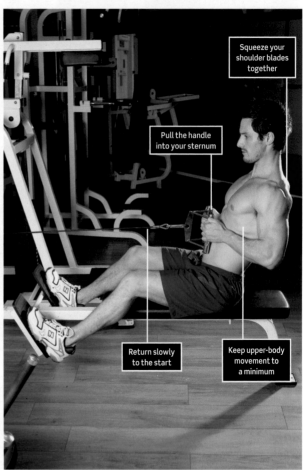

Squeeze your shoulder blades together

Pull the handle into your sternum

Return slowly to the start

Keep upper-body movement to a minimum

Variations

WIDE-GRIP CABLE ROW

Place more emphasis on your rear deltoids (back of your shoulders) and mid traps.

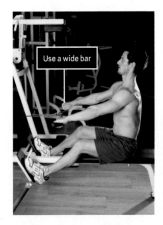

Use a wide bar

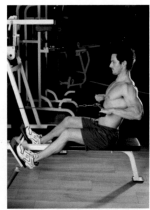

SQUAT-TO-ROW

This turns the cable row into a full-body movement that works the legs, core, back and shoulders.

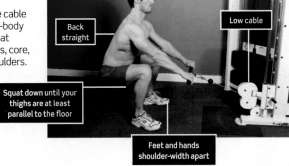

Back straight

Low cable

Squat down until your thighs are at least parallel to the floor

Feet and hands shoulder-width apart

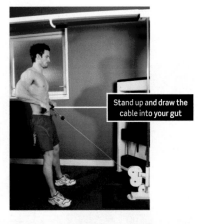

Stand up and draw the cable into your gut

INVERTED ROW

Use your own body weight to complete the row.

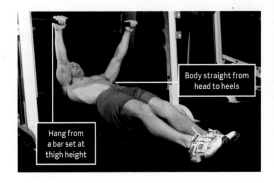

Body straight from head to heels

Hang from a bar set at thigh height

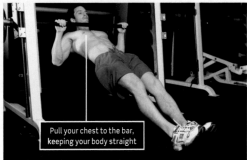

Pull your chest to the bar, keeping your body straight

One-arm row

Target: **traps, lats, rhomboids**

Work each side of your back independently while pulling heavy weights.

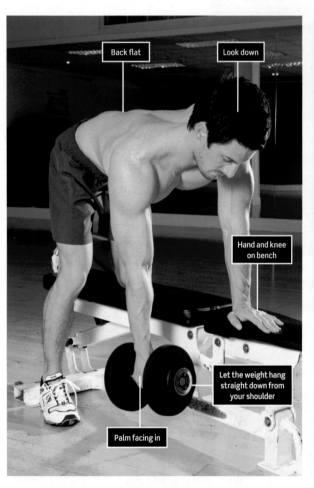

Back flat

Look down

Hand and knee on bench

Let the weight hang straight down from your shoulder

Palm facing in

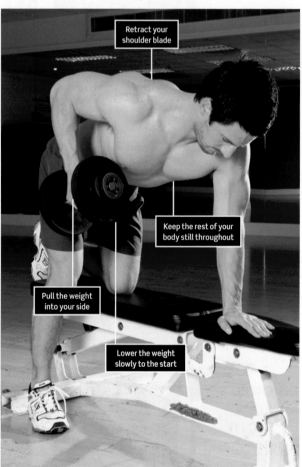

Retract your shoulder blade

Keep the rest of your body still throughout

Pull the weight into your side

Lower the weight slowly to the start

Variations

ONE-ARM REVERSE FLYE

The flye movement takes the arm muscles out of the equation and places all the stress on the traps and rear deltoids.

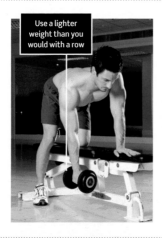

Use a lighter weight than you would with a row

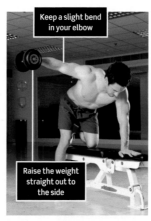

Keep a slight bend in your elbow

Raise the weight straight out to the side

ONE-ARM CABLE ROW

Give your core a workout by holding your body upright during the row. This takes some of the stress off the lats and places it on the rear deltoid.

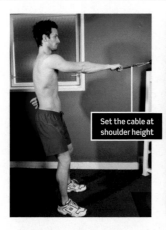

Set the cable at shoulder height

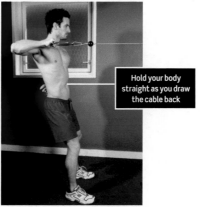

Hold your body straight as you draw the cable back

SPLIT SQUAT TO ONE-ARM ROW

This whole-body move works the legs, back, arms and shoulders, and introduces a rotational effect to work your core muscles.

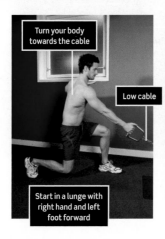

Turn your body towards the cable

Low cable

Start in a lunge with right hand and left foot forward

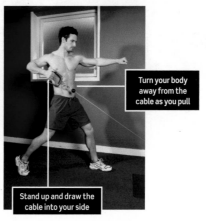

Turn your body away from the cable as you pull

Stand up and draw the cable into your side

Pull-up

Target: lats, traps, rhomboids

Work against your own body weight in this classic test of strength. The overhand grip ensures most of the work is done by your back and not your arms.

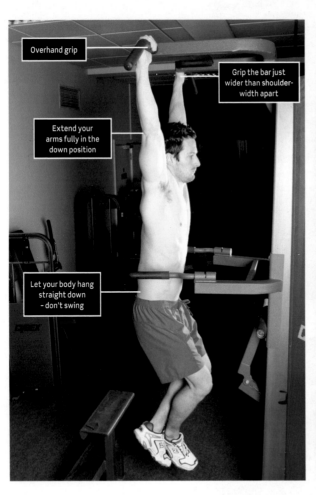

Overhand grip

Grip the bar just wider than shoulder-width apart

Extend your arms fully in the down position

Let your body hang straight down – don't swing

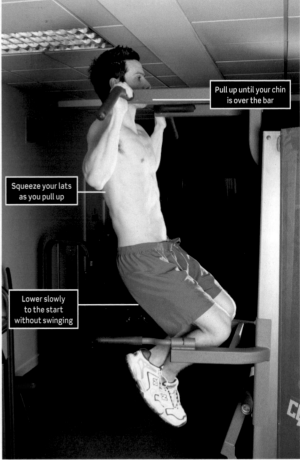

Pull up until your chin is over the bar

Squeeze your lats as you pull up

Lower slowly to the start without swinging

Variations

NEGATIVE PULL-UP

Use a bench or a helper to get yourself into the 'up' position and then lower yourself as slowly as you can. This lets you do a few more reps after failure and stimulates the eccentric muscle growth.

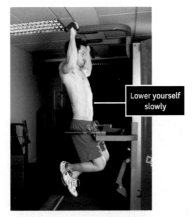

Lower yourself slowly

WEIGHTED PULL-UP

If you can do lots of pull-ups, a weight belt will make sure that you hit failure within your chosen rep range.

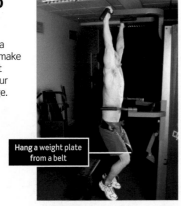

Hang a weight plate from a belt

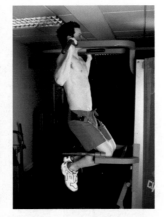

WIDE-GRIP PULL-UP

Place greater emphasis on your lats by widening your grip. It makes the movement shorter but tougher.

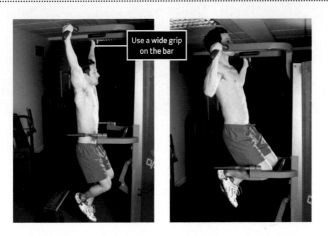

Use a wide grip on the bar

Lat pull-down

Target: **lats, traps, rhomboids**
Works similar muscle groups to the wide-grip
pull-up, but allows you to adjust the resistance easily.

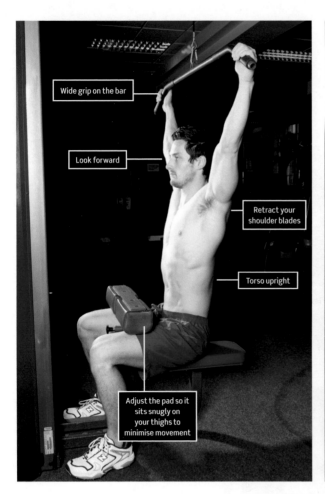

Wide grip on the bar

Look forward

Retract your
shoulder blades

Torso upright

Adjust the pad so it
sits snugly on
your thighs to
minimise movement

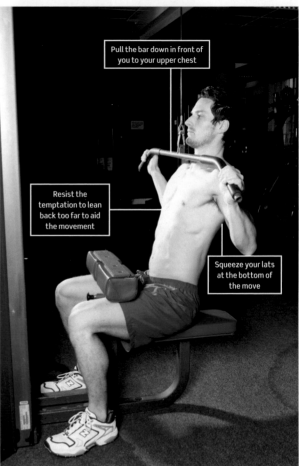

Pull the bar down in front of
you to your upper chest

Resist the
temptation to lean
back too far to aid
the movement

Squeeze your lats
at the bottom of
the move

Variations

UNILATERAL LAT PULL-DOWN

Work one side of your body at a time for balanced gains.

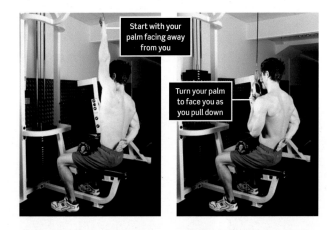

Start with your palm facing away from you

Turn your palm to face you as you pull down

CLOSE-GRIP LAT PULL-DOWN TO TRICEPS PRESS-DOWN

Turn a lats move into a triceps move in a single exercise.

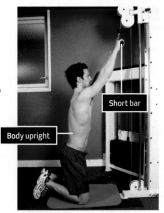

Short bar

Body upright

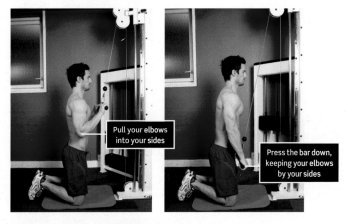

Pull your elbows into your sides

Press the bar down, keeping your elbows by your sides

STRAIGHT-ARM PULL-DOWN

Focus on your lats with this single-joint move.

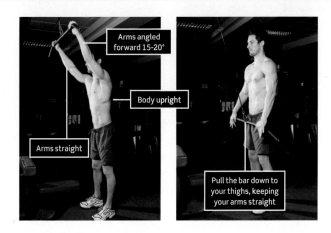

Arms angled forward 15-20°

Body upright

Arms straight

Pull the bar down to your thighs, keeping your arms straight

Shrug

Target: **upper traps**
Go heavy to build a powerful upper back.

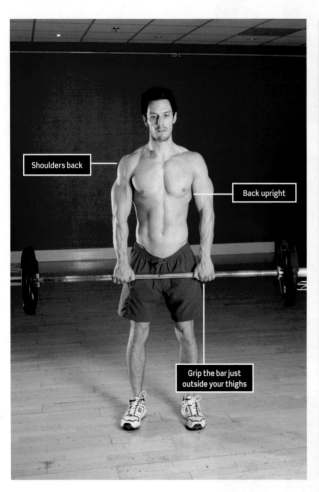

Shoulders back

Back upright

Grip the bar just outside your thighs

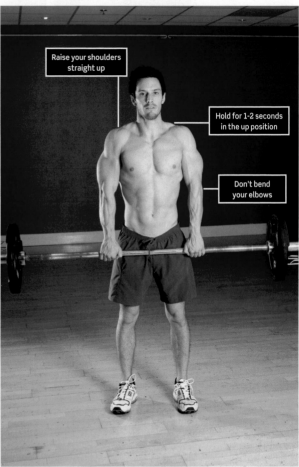

Raise your shoulders straight up

Hold for 1-2 seconds in the up position

Don't bend your elbows

Variations

UPRIGHT ROW

Bring your shoulders into play to aid your upper traps in lifting the weight.

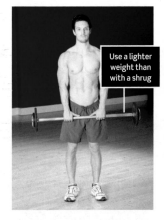

Use a lighter weight than with a shrug

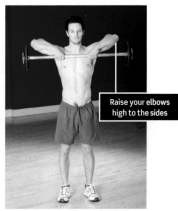

Raise your elbows high to the sides

DUMB-BELL SHRUG

Using dumb-bells allows you hold your hands in a more comfortable position at your sides, and works both sides of the body independently.

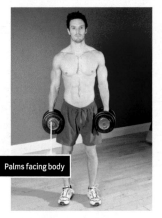

Palms facing body

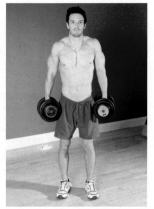

DUMB-BELL UPRIGHT ROW AND SHRUG

Combine the row and shrug to give your upper traps a double hit.

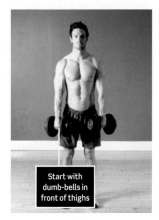

Start with dumb-bells in front of thighs

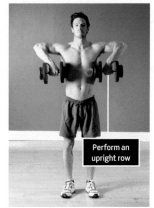

Perform an upright row

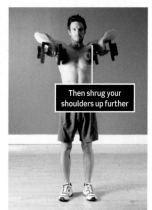

Then shrug your shoulders up further

Good morning

Target: lower back, hamstrings, glutes

This move will strengthen your erector spinae muscles as well as the backs of your legs. Be sure to maintain perfect form to prevent injuries.

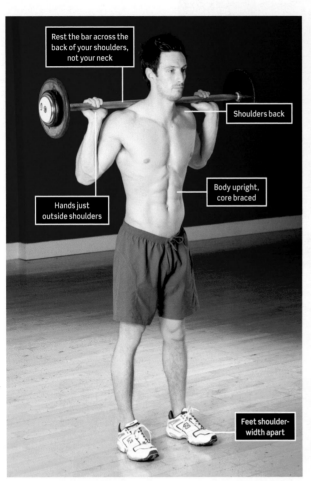

Rest the bar across the back of your shoulders, not your neck

Shoulders back

Body upright, core braced

Hands just outside shoulders

Feet shoulder-width apart

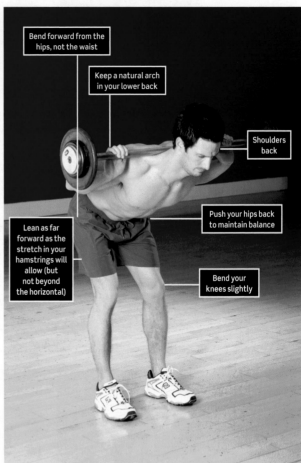

Bend forward from the hips, not the waist

Keep a natural arch in your lower back

Shoulders back

Push your hips back to maintain balance

Lean as far forward as the stretch in your hamstrings will allow (but not beyond the horizontal)

Bend your knees slightly

Variations

SPLIT GOOD MORNING
Place extra pressure on your hamstrings with this one-sided move.

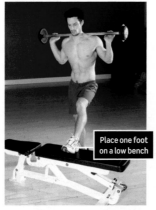 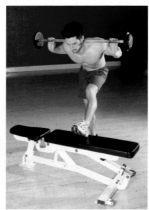

Place one foot on a low bench

SINGLE-LEG GOOD MORNING
Standing on one leg requires your core muscles – lower back and abdominals – to work harder to maintain balance.

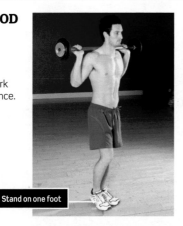 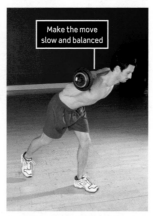

Make the move slow and balanced

Stand on one foot

MEDICINE-BALL SLEDGEHAMMER
Done quickly and powerfully, this exercise targets a host of muscles around your body, especially the stabilising muscles in your lower back.

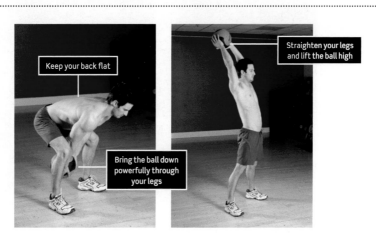

Keep your back flat

Straighten your legs and lift the ball high

Bring the ball down powerfully through your legs

Two-point box

Target: **lower back**

This simple move will strengthen the stabilising muscles around your spine, which will help to keep you strong and injury-free when doing bigger lifts.

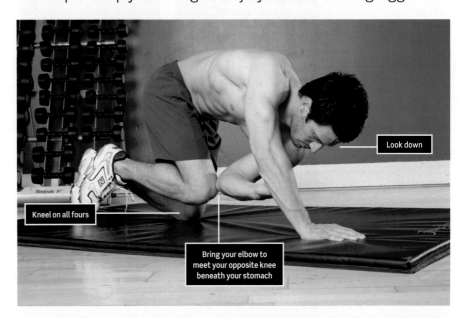

Look down

Kneel on all fours

Bring your elbow to meet your opposite knee beneath your stomach

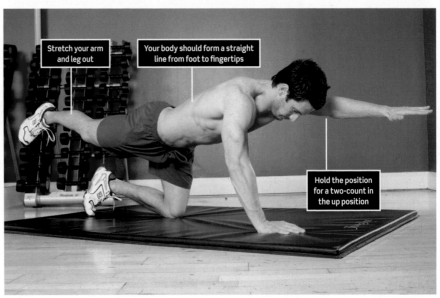

Stretch your arm and leg out

Your body should form a straight line from foot to fingertips

Hold the position for a two-count in the up position

Variations

DORSAL RAISE WITH SHOULDER ROTATION

Twisting your hands back at the top of the move squeezes your shoulder blades together for a stronger contraction.

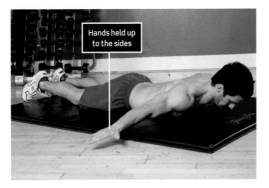

Hands held up to the sides

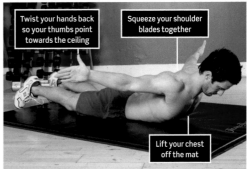

Twist your hands back so your thumbs point towards the ceiling

Squeeze your shoulder blades together

Lift your chest off the mat

AQUAMAN

The swimming motion is not as easy as it looks and is great for a strong lower back.

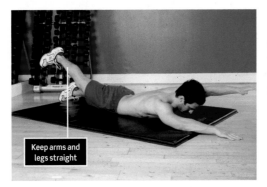

Keep arms and legs straight

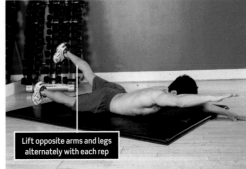

Lift opposite arms and legs alternately with each rep

SWISS BALL BACK EXTENSION

The ball allows for a greater range of motion when exercising your lower back.

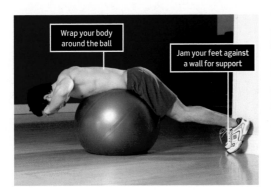

Wrap your body around the ball

Jam your feet against a wall for support

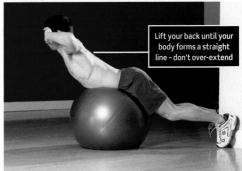

Lift your back until your body forms a straight line – don't over-extend

CHEST

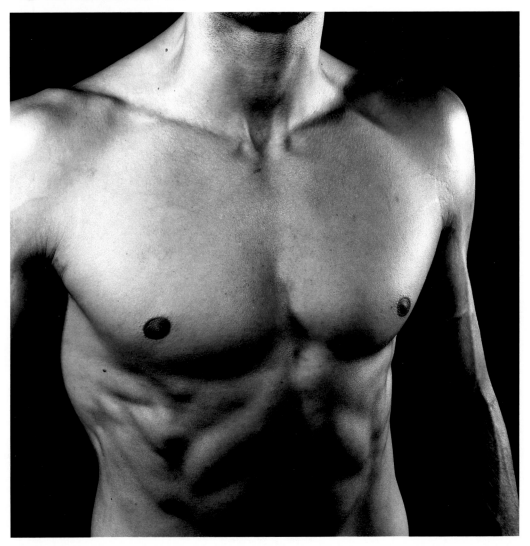

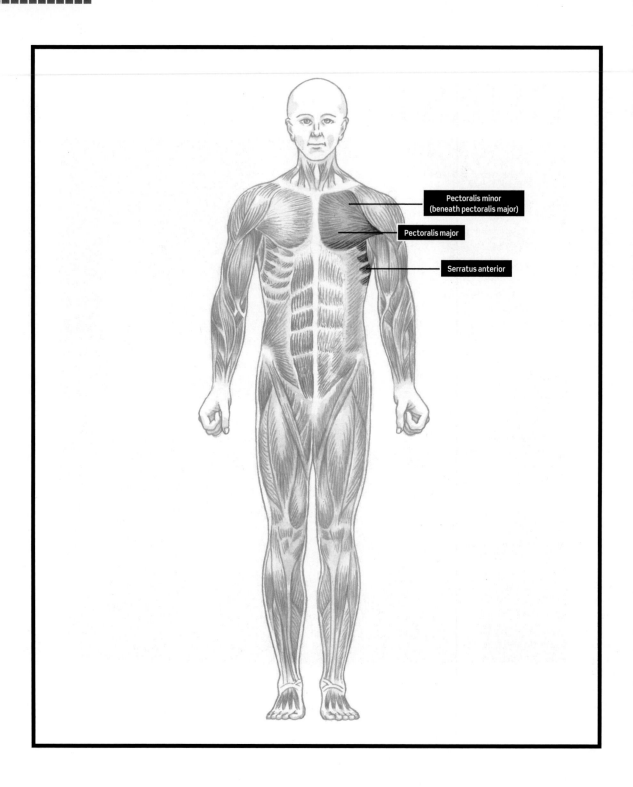

Pectoralis minor
(beneath pectoralis major)

Pectoralis major

Serratus anterior

CHEST

You mostly use your chest muscles (pectorals) when you push objects away from you. So the most obvious exercise to build up your chest is the bench press. In this you use your pectorals, serratus, front shoulders and triceps to press a heavy bar directly above your chest from a lying position.

The bench press has long been considered the main test of upper-body strength for men, which is why every gym has a queue for the bench press rack, and why a certain type of gym-goer always opens every conversation with the question: 'So, what do you bench?'

Despite the undisputed benefits of the bench press – you should make it the cornerstone of your chest workout – be wary of focusing on this one exercise at the expense of all others. Like any muscles, the pecs need to be worked from a variety of angles to get the maximum growth stimulation, and simply changing the angle of the bench, or opting for dumb-bells instead of a barbell, can make a world of difference to the development of your chest.

The pectoralis major is a large block of muscle that attaches to your ribs beneath the collarbone. Although it is one single muscle, training experience suggests you can target the upper, middle or lower portions of your chest muscle depending on the angle from which you attack it. An incline bench press will focus most of the effort on the upper portion of your pecs, for example, although it will still work the entire pectoral muscle.

Main exercises

Bench press	94
Dumb-bell bench press	96
Incline bench press	98
Decline bench press	100
Dumb-bell flye	102
T press-up	104
Dumb-bell pullover	106

Bench press

Target: pecs

This staple of most men's workouts is still the
best way to build a powerful chest.

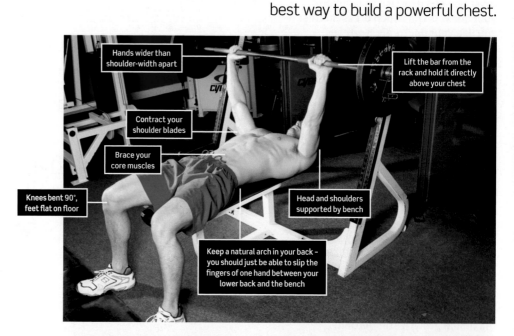

Hands wider than
shoulder-width apart

Lift the bar from the
rack and hold it directly
above your chest

Contract your
shoulder blades

Brace your
core muscles

Knees bent 90°,
feet flat on floor

Head and shoulders
supported by bench

Keep a natural arch in your back –
you should just be able to slip the
fingers of one hand between your
lower back and the bench

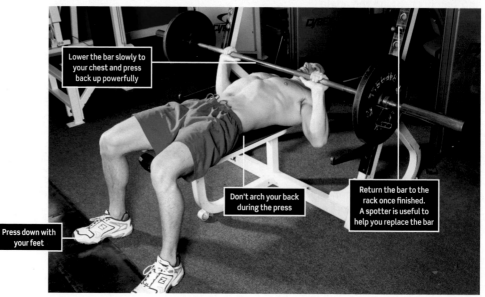

Lower the bar slowly to
your chest and press
back up powerfully

Don't arch your back
during the press

Return the bar to the
rack once finished.
A spotter is useful to
help you replace the bar

Press down with
your feet

Variations

BALLISTIC BENCH PRESS

Push the bar up explosively, as if you were trying to throw it off you, to fire up your fast-twitch muscle fibres (just don't let go!).

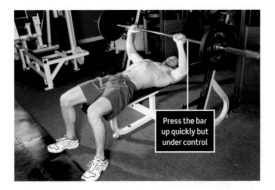

Press the bar up quickly but under control

SMITH MACHINE PRESS

The machine locks the bar into a path so you can concentrate on pressing the maximum weight in safety.

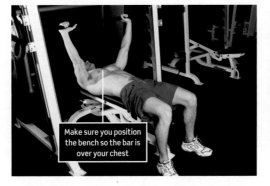

Make sure you position the bench so the bar is over your chest

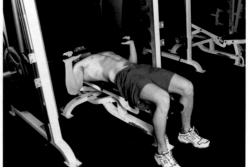

PRESS-UP

Work your chest anywhere, any time with this simple, classic move.

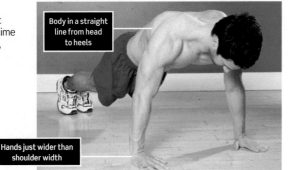

Body in a straight line from head to heels

Hands just wider than shoulder width

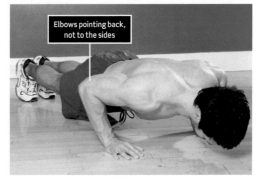

Elbows pointing back, not to the sides

Dumb-bell bench press

Target: **pecs**

Dumb-bells take more effort to stabilise than a bar, and allow for a greater range of movement, making the move tougher.

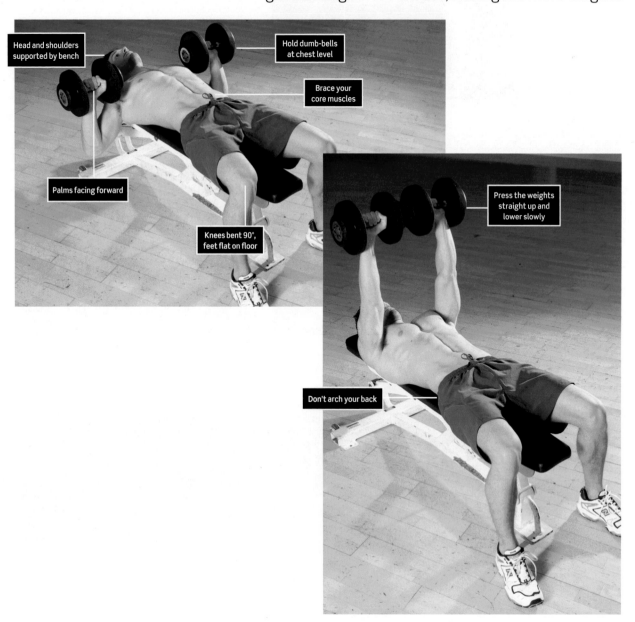

Head and shoulders supported by bench

Hold dumb-bells at chest level

Brace your core muscles

Palms facing forward

Knees bent 90°, feet flat on floor

Press the weights straight up and lower slowly

Don't arch your back

Variations

SWISS BALL DUMB-BELL PRESS

Lying on a Swiss ball means you have to stabilise your entire body, which helps to build a stronger foundation from which to improve your bench presses.

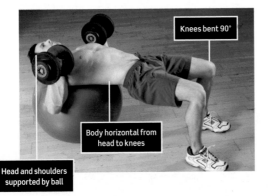
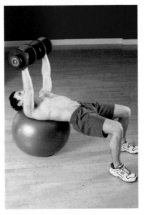

Knees bent 90°

Body horizontal from head to knees

Head and shoulders supported by ball

ALTERNATING DUMB-BELL PRESS

Work each side of your chest independently to iron out any muscle imbalances.

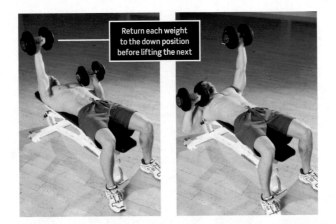

Return each weight to the down position before lifting the next

SWISS BALL PRESS-UP

This deceptively difficult move requires your chest muscles to control the wobble, making them more stable in heavier presses.

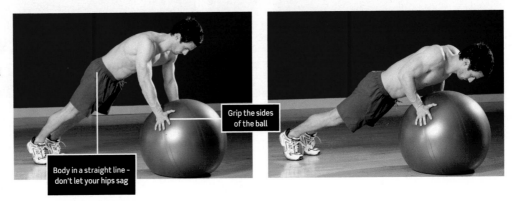

Grip the sides of the ball

Body in a straight line – don't let your hips sag

Incline bench press

Target: **upper pecs**

Place the focus on the upper part of your chest by tilting the bench upwards.

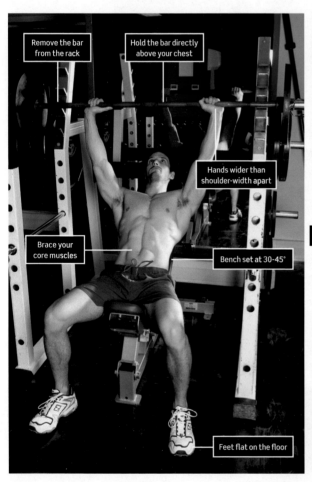

Remove the bar from the rack

Hold the bar directly above your chest

Hands wider than shoulder-width apart

Brace your core muscles

Bench set at 30-45°

Feet flat on the floor

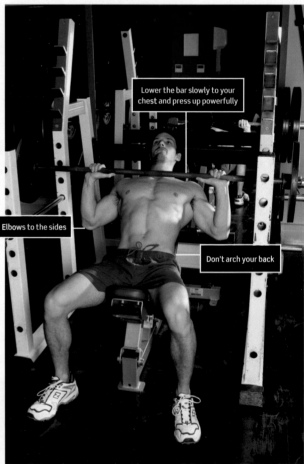

Lower the bar slowly to your chest and press up powerfully

Elbows to the sides

Don't arch your back

Variations

SWISS BALL DECLINE PRESS-UP

The additional wobble gives your core a good workout as well as your upper chest, shoulders and triceps.

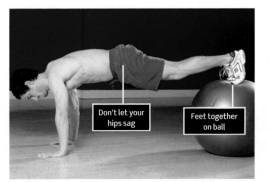

Don't let your hips sag

Feet together on ball

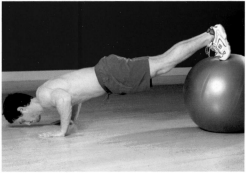

INCLINE DUMB-BELL PRESS

Work both sides of your chest independently to prevent your stronger side doing all the work.

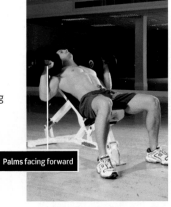

Palms facing forward

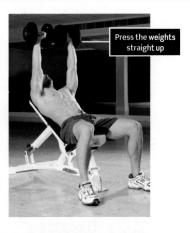

Press the weights straight up

INCLINE SMITH MACHINE PRESS

When you don't have a spotter to help you, the Smith machine lets you press heavy weights in safety.

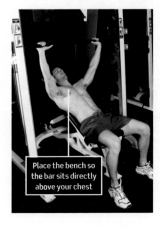

Place the bench so the bar sits directly above your chest

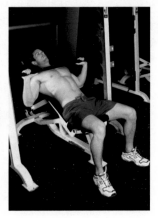

Decline bench press

Target: lower pecs

By angling the bench downwards you target the lower portion of your chest.

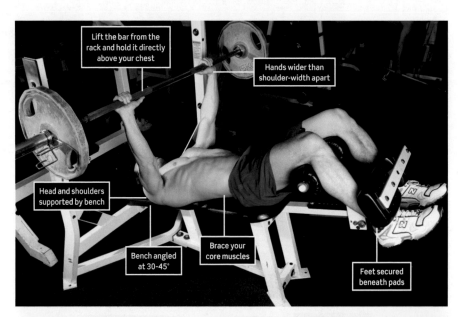

Lift the bar from the rack and hold it directly above your chest

Hands wider than shoulder-width apart

Head and shoulders supported by bench

Bench angled at 30-45°

Brace your core muscles

Feet secured beneath pads

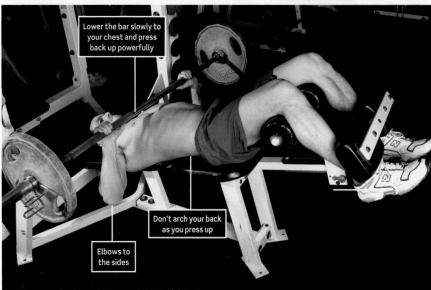

Lower the bar slowly to your chest and press back up powerfully

Don't arch your back as you press up

Elbows to the sides

Variations

INCLINE PRESS-UP

A great way to warm up before doing decline presses, or to exhaust your lower pec muscles safely afterwards.

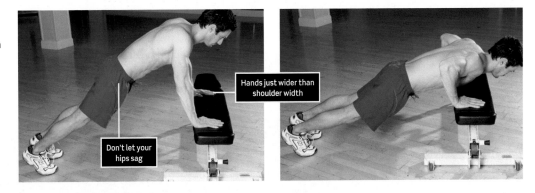

Hands just wider than shoulder width

Don't let your hips sag

DECLINE DUMB-BELL PRESS

The dumb-bells allow for a greater range of motion than the bar, and can be kinder to your shoulder and elbow joints.

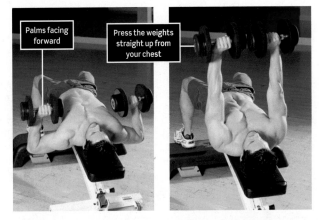

Palms facing forward

Press the weights straight up from your chest

DECLINE SMITH MACHINE PRESS

The Smith machine means you don't have to worry about controlling the bar, so you can afford to go as heavy as you dare.

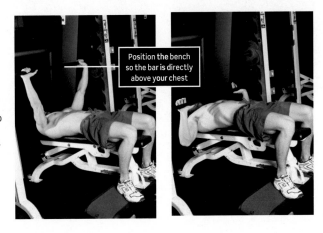

Position the bench so the bar is directly above your chest

Dumb-bell flye

Target: pecs

The flye isolates your chest by taking your arm muscles out of the equation.

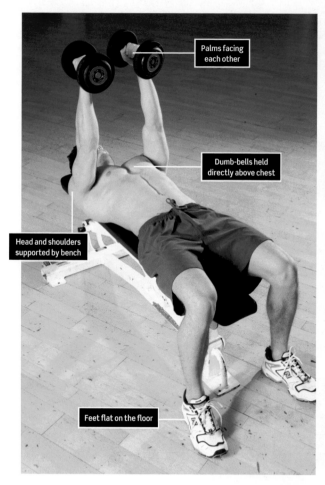

Palms facing each other

Dumb-bells held directly above chest

Head and shoulders supported by bench

Feet flat on the floor

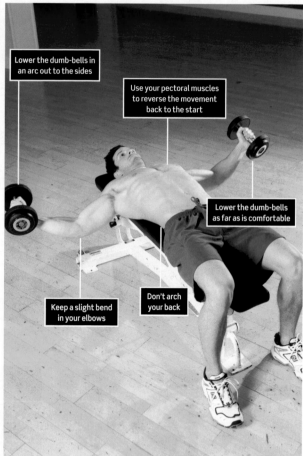

Lower the dumb-bells in an arc out to the sides

Use your pectoral muscles to reverse the movement back to the start

Lower the dumb-bells as far as is comfortable

Keep a slight bend in your elbows

Don't arch your back

Variations

SWISS BALL DUMB-BELL FLYE

The ball requires you to hold your body rigid during the move, ensuring that you use good form to execute the flye.

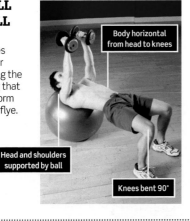

Body horizontal from head to knees

Head and shoulders supported by ball

Knees bent 90°

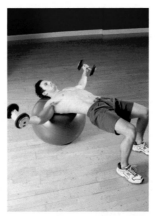

INCLINE DUMB-BELL FLYE

Place the emphasis on your upper pecs by tilting the bench upwards.

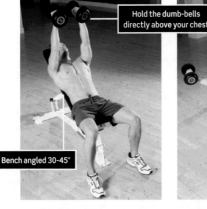

Hold the dumb-bells directly above your chest

Bench angled 30-45°

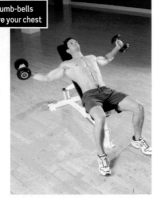

CABLE CROSSOVER

The cables give greater resistance than dumb-bells at the point where your hands come together, creating a powerful contraction in your pectorals.

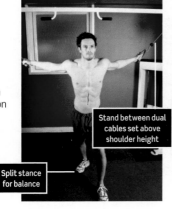

Stand between dual cables set above shoulder height

Split stance for balance

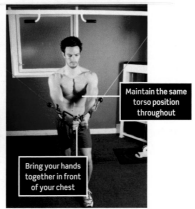

Maintain the same torso position throughout

Bring your hands together in front of your chest

T press-up

Target: pecs

Turn the humble press-up into a powerful muscle-building tool that works the chest, shoulders, arms and core in one dynamic move.

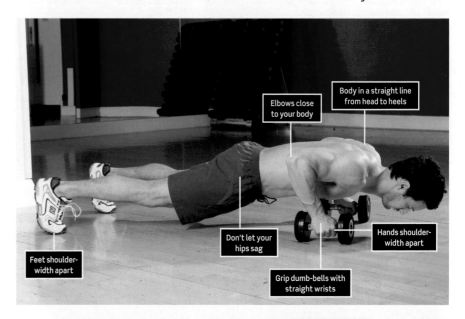

Body in a straight line from head to heels

Elbows close to your body

Hands shoulder-width apart

Don't let your hips sag

Grip dumb-bells with straight wrists

Feet shoulder-width apart

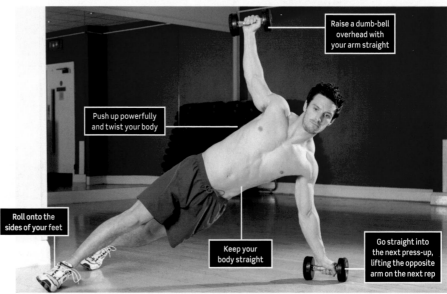

Raise a dumb-bell overhead with your arm straight

Push up powerfully and twist your body

Roll onto the sides of your feet

Keep your body straight

Go straight into the next press-up, lifting the opposite arm on the next rep

Variations

CLAP PRESS-UP

When you push up explosively enough so that you can clap your hands, you target the fast-twitch muscle fibres that have the most potential for growth.

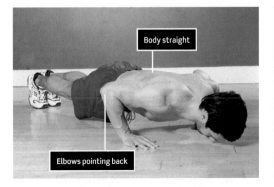

Body straight

Elbows pointing back

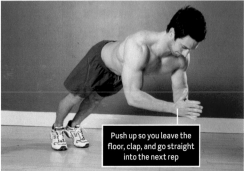

Push up so you leave the floor, clap, and go straight into the next rep

PASSING MEDICINE-BALL PRESS-UP

This move blends power and co-ordination to give you functional upper-body strength.

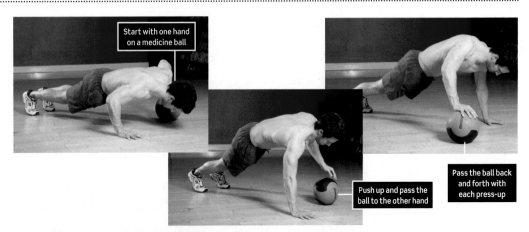

Start with one hand on a medicine ball

Push up and pass the ball to the other hand

Pass the ball back and forth with each press-up

ALTERNATING OFFSET JUMP PRESS-UP

Jump your hands backwards and forwards while doing shallow press-ups to hit your muscles from different angles.

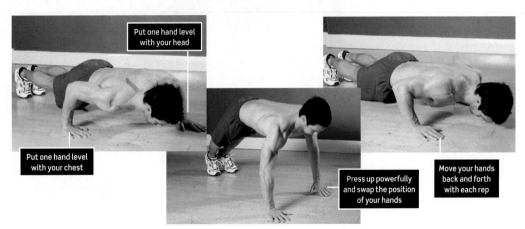

Put one hand level with your head

Put one hand level with your chest

Press up powerfully and swap the position of your hands

Move your hands back and forth with each rep

Dumb-bell pullover

Target: **pecs, lats**

An single-joint move that hits your lower chest, lats and triceps.

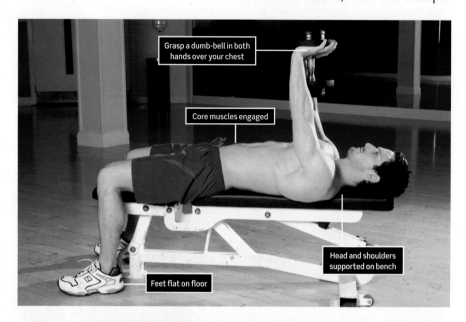

Grasp a dumb-bell in both hands over your chest

Core muscles engaged

Head and shoulders supported on bench

Feet flat on floor

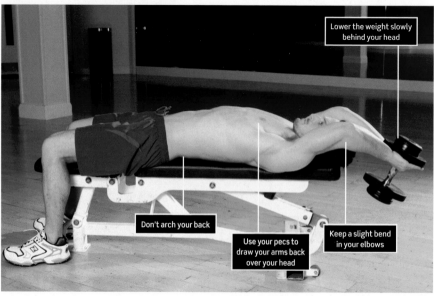

Lower the weight slowly behind your head

Don't arch your back

Use your pecs to draw your arms back over your head

Keep a slight bend in your elbows

Variations

SWISS BALL DUMB-BELL PULLOVER

Counteracting the wobble gives your core a thorough workout as well as your chest.

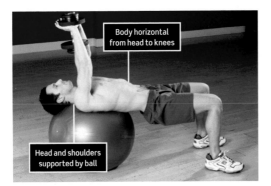

Body horizontal from head to knees

Head and shoulders supported by ball

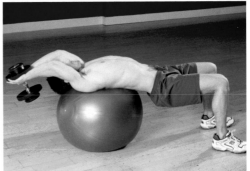

DUMB-BELL PULLOVER PRESS

By bending your elbows and straightening them as you raise the weight, you give your triceps and extra workout.

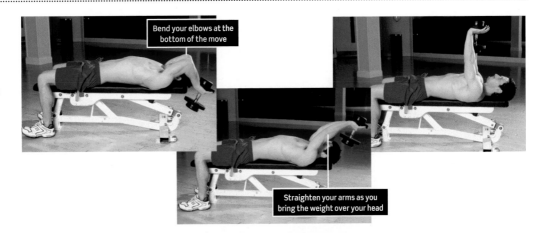

Bend your elbows at the bottom of the move

Straighten your arms as you bring the weight over your head

CABLE PULLOVER

The cable ensures that you don't lose resistance at the top of the move.

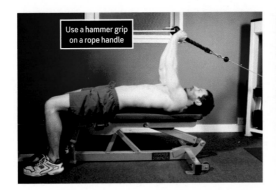

Use a hammer grip on a rope handle

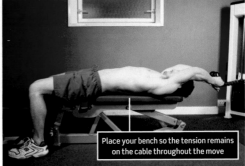

Place your bench so the tension remains on the cable throughout the move

LEGS

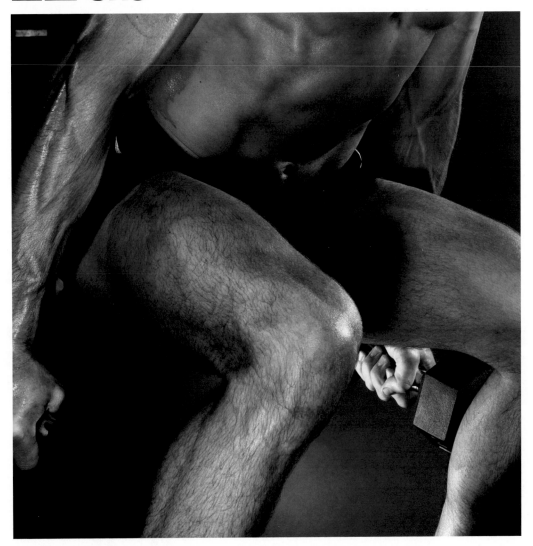

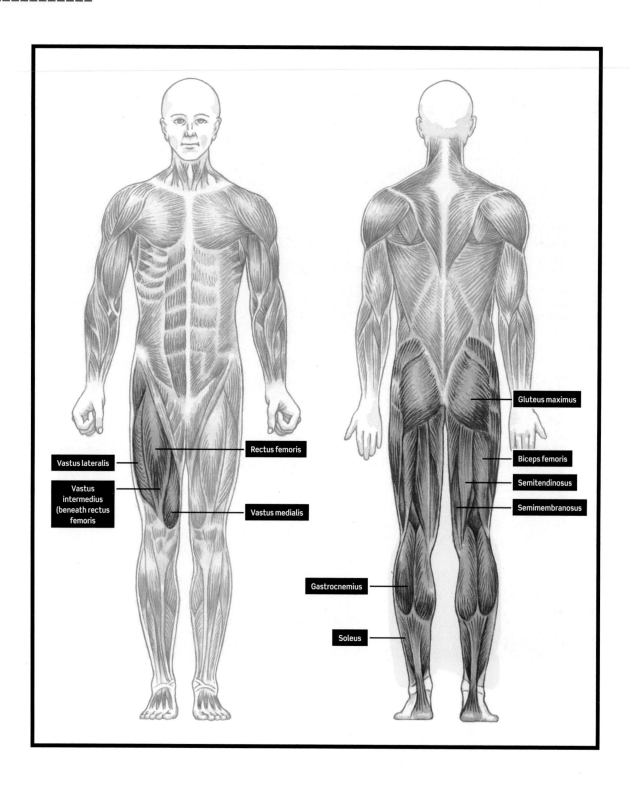

Vastus lateralis

Rectus femoris

Vastus intermedius (beneath rectus femoris

Vastus medialis

Gluteus maximus

Biceps femoris

Semitendinosus

Semimembranosus

Gastrocnemius

Soleus

LEGS

Your legs and backside (glutes) contain the biggest muscles in your body and form half of your total muscle mass, but do you give them half of your workout time? Too many gym-goers relegate legs to occasional workout sessions, which explains the popularity of long shorts on the beach. But what's the point of having bulging biceps and a huge chest if they sit atop a pair of sparrow legs? A *Men's Fitness* survey discovered that the part of a man that women most liked to stare at is the bum, so you've no excuse for ignoring your lower half.

What's more, if you want to build big muscles in your upper half, you need to work the muscles of your lower half. The reason is that the leg muscles are so large that training them creates a huge hormonal surge in your body that affects all your muscles – so doing squats can help you to build your biceps.

The main muscles on the front of your thighs are the quadriceps. As the name suggests they are made up of four heads that help to straighten your knee and stabilise your kneecap. On the back of your thighs the hamstrings are mainly concerned with extending your hips and flexing your knee. Together, your quads and hams work with your glutes every time you go from a sitting to a standing position.

To build muscle mass on your legs, no exercise is more effective than the squat. You are obliged to move heavy weights while stabilising your body, and the move involves a huge number of lower body muscle fibres. For many people the squat can seem like a tricky move, but it's worth practising to ensure perfect form. Once you've got it, it will form the cornerstone of your muscle-building workouts. Using a Smith machine can help to stabilise your body if you are worried about maintaining good form with heavy weights, but it should not be seen as a replacement for good squat technique.

Having said that, as always you should do as wide a variety of leg exercises as possible to keep your muscles guessing – and growing.

Main exercises

Squat	112
Smith squat	114
Front squat	116
Dumb-bell step-up	118
Lunge	120
Lateral lunge	122
Bulgarian split squat	124
Romanian deadlift	126
Swiss ball leg curl	128
Standing calf raise	130

Squat

Target: quads, glutes, hamstrings

The king of all leg exercises, this uses many different muscle groups and should be in every man's mass-building arsenal.

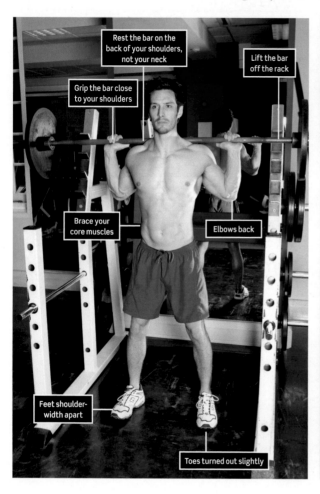

Rest the bar on the back of your shoulders, not your neck

Lift the bar off the rack

Grip the bar close to your shoulders

Brace your core muscles

Elbows back

Feet shoulder-width apart

Toes turned out slightly

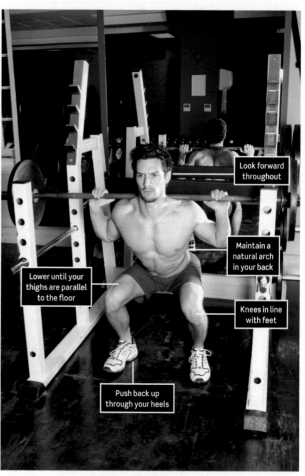

Look forward throughout

Maintain a natural arch in your back

Knees in line with feet

Lower until your thighs are parallel to the floor

Push back up through your heels

Variations

DUMB-BELL SQUAT

If you struggle to maintain good form with a barbell, dumb-bells can help you to learn the move safely.

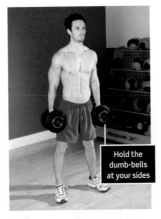

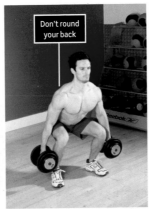

Don't round your back

Hold the dumb-bells at your sides

JUMP SQUAT

Add an explosive element to the squat to develop your fast-twitch muscle fibres – just remember to keep the weight light.

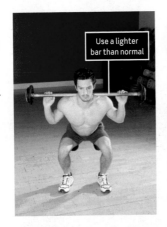

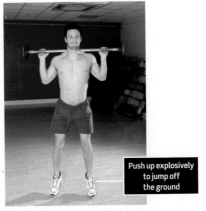

Use a lighter bar than normal

Push up explosively to jump off the ground

ONE-LEG SQUAT

Develops balance and co-ordination, as well as strengthening the muscles that stabilise your knees and ankles.

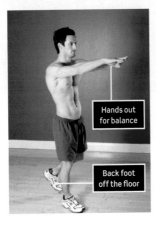

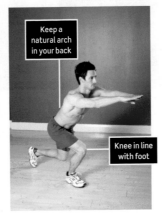

Hands out for balance

Back foot off the floor

Keep a natural arch in your back

Knee in line with foot

Smith squat

Target: quads

The Smith machine allows you to press more weight without worrying about controlling the bar.

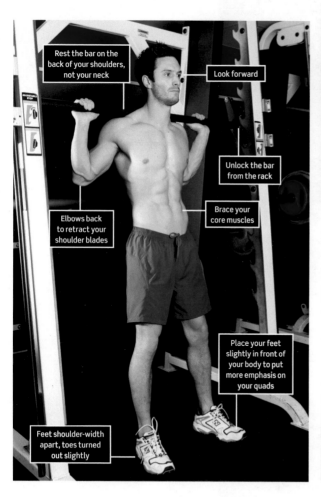

Rest the bar on the back of your shoulders, not your neck

Look forward

Unlock the bar from the rack

Elbows back to retract your shoulder blades

Brace your core muscles

Place your feet slightly in front of your body to put more emphasis on your quads

Feet shoulder-width apart, toes turned out slightly

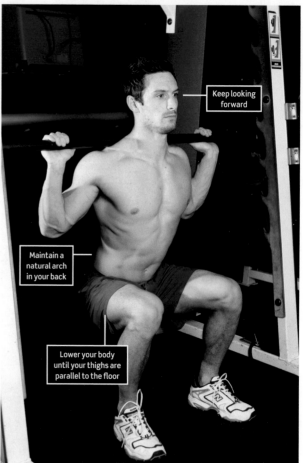

Keep looking forward

Maintain a natural arch in your back

Lower your body until your thighs are parallel to the floor

Variations

ONE-LEG SMITH SQUAT

Work each leg independently to iron out any muscle imbalances.

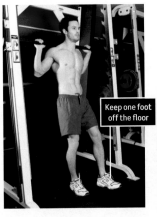
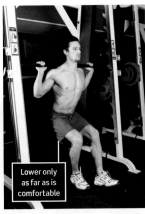

Keep one foot off the floor

Lower only as far as is comfortable

DUMB-BELL SWISS BALL SQUAT

If you don't have access to a Smith machine, this is a suitable alternative, and it forces your core to work harder to control the motion.

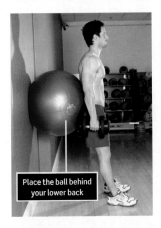
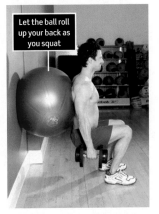

Let the ball roll up your back as you squat

Place the ball behind your lower back

STATIC SKI SQUAT

Feel the burn in your quads by holding this isometric position for as long as you can.

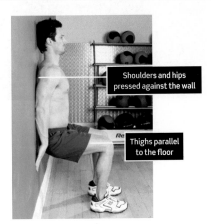

Shoulders and hips pressed against the wall

Thighs parallel to the floor

Front squat

Target: quads

Placing the bar on the front of your shoulders makes your back more upright in the squat, emphasising your quads and lessening the pressure on your lower back.

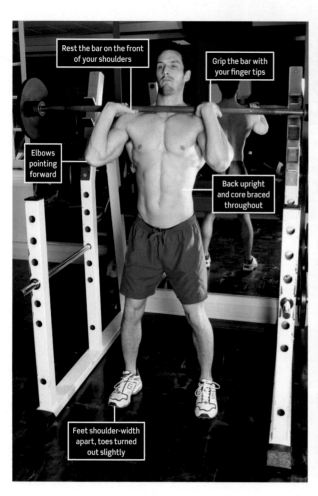

Rest the bar on the front of your shoulders

Grip the bar with your finger tips

Elbows pointing forward

Back upright and core braced throughout

Feet shoulder-width apart, toes turned out slightly

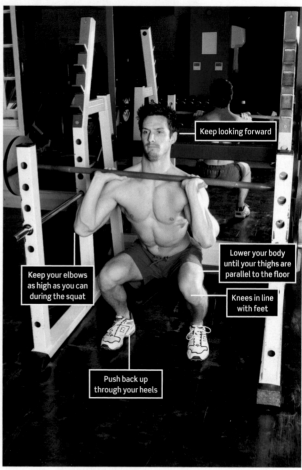

Keep looking forward

Keep your elbows as high as you can during the squat

Lower your body until your thighs are parallel to the floor

Knees in line with feet

Push back up through your heels

Variations

OVERHEAD SQUAT

A difficult move that tests your posture and shoulder mobility to the full.

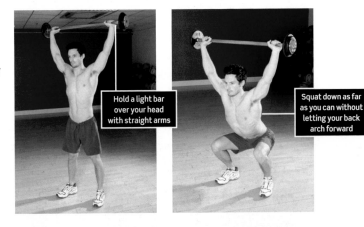

Hold a light bar over your head with straight arms

Squat down as far as you can without letting your back arch forward

SUMO SQUAT

Take a wide stance to alter the effect on your quads. More emphasis will be placed on the inner thigh.

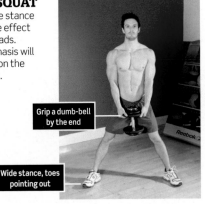

Grip a dumb-bell by the end

Wide stance, toes pointing out

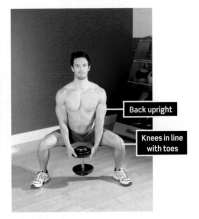

Back upright

Knees in line with toes

CROSS-GRIP FRONT SQUAT

Folding your arms provides a platform for the bar to rest on the front of your shoulders. This is useful for people who find the front squat places strain on their shoulder joints.

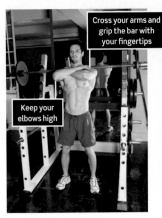

Cross your arms and grip the bar with your fingertips

Keep your elbows high

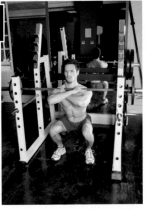

Dumb-bell step-up

Target: glutes, quads

It's a move you do every day when climbing stairs, so this exercise provides functional strength.

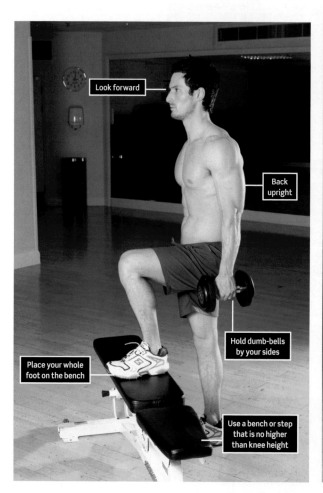

Look forward

Back upright

Hold dumb-bells by your sides

Place your whole foot on the bench

Use a bench or step that is no higher than knee height

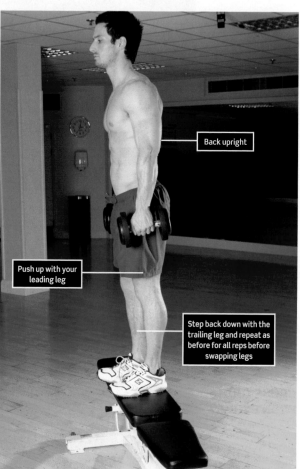

Back upright

Push up with your leading leg

Step back down with the trailing leg and repeat as before for all reps before swapping legs

Variations

ONE-LEG BENCH SQUAT

Focus on your quads and the muscles that stabilise your knees.

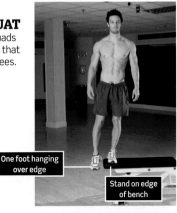

One foot hanging over edge

Stand on edge of bench

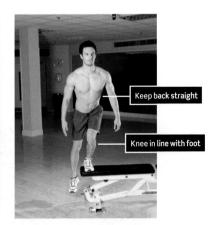

Keep back straight

Knee in line with foot

SIDE STEP-UP

Attack your glutes from a new angle, introducing your inner-thigh muscles (adductors) to help with the workload.

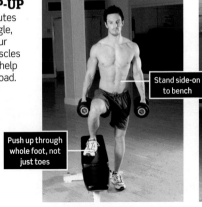

Stand side-on to bench

Push up through whole foot, not just toes

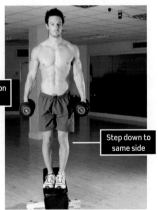

Step down to same side

STEP-UP AND JUMP

Improve sporting prowess with a plyometric move that builds power in your glutes and quads.

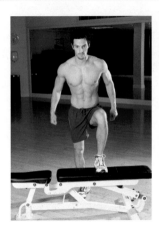

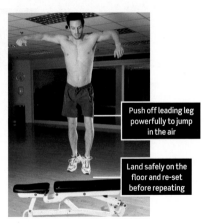

Push off leading leg powerfully to jump in the air

Land safely on the floor and re-set before repeating

Lunge

Target: **quads, hamstrings,**
This classic move requires both power and co-ordination, both of which are vital for sports.

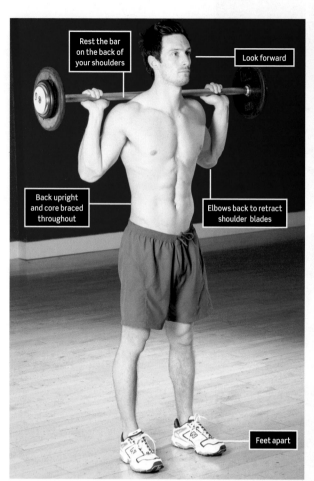

Rest the bar on the back of your shoulders

Look forward

Back upright and core braced throughout

Elbows back to retract shoulder blades

Feet apart

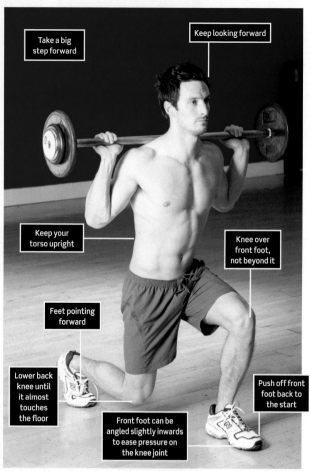

Take a big step forward

Keep looking forward

Keep your torso upright

Knee over front foot, not beyond it

Feet pointing forward

Lower back knee until it almost touches the floor

Push off front foot back to the start

Front foot can be angled slightly inwards to ease pressure on the knee joint

Variations

SPLIT SQUAT

It's like a lunge but without the initial step, so you can ensure that your form is perfect and take some of the pressure off your knees.

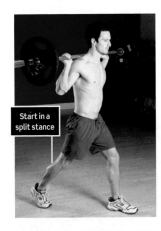

Start in a split stance

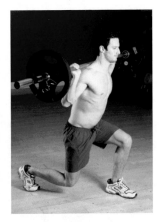

JUMPING LUNGE

From a lunge, jump up and land in another lunge. This move is great for functional power and stability.

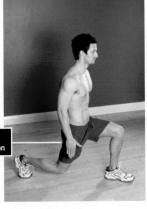

Start in a lunge position

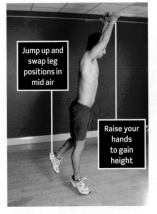

Jump up and swap leg positions in mid air

Raise your hands to gain height

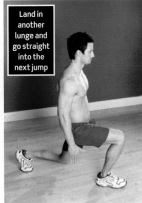

Land in another lunge and go straight into the next jump

REVERSE LUNGE

By stepping backwards instead of forwards you place a slightly different stress on your quads and hams. It also promotes good co-ordination.

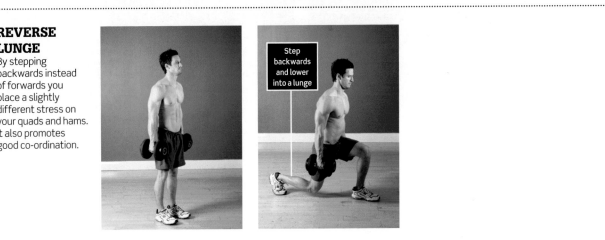

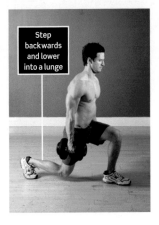

Step backwards and lower into a lunge

Lateral lunge

Target: adductors

All too often ignored, your inner thighs are vital in turning movements during sport.

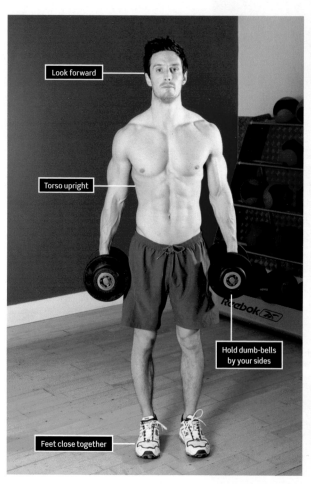

- Look forward
- Torso upright
- Hold dumb-bells by your sides
- Feet close together

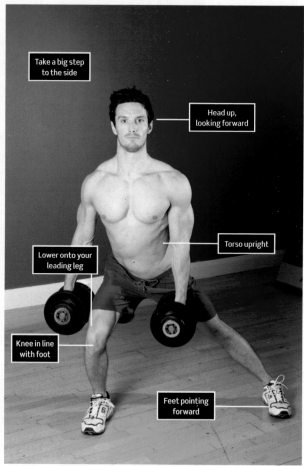

- Take a big step to the side
- Head up, looking forward
- Torso upright
- Lower onto your leading leg
- Knee in line with foot
- Feet pointing forward

Variations

TRANSVERSE LUNGE

Open up your hips to perform this move, which will help you to turn quickly at sports without damaging your groin.

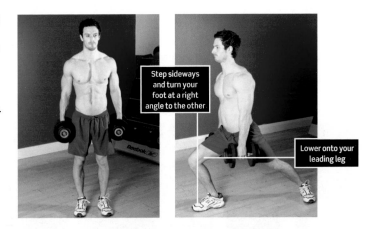

Step sideways and turn your foot at a right angle to the other

Lower onto your leading leg

DUMB-BELL LATERAL LUNGE AND TOUCH

Work your hamstrings in conjunction with your quads and adductors in this multi-joint move.

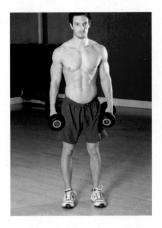

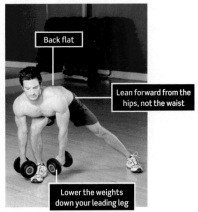

Back flat

Lean forward from the hips, not the waist

Lower the weights down your leading leg

CABLE LATERAL LUNGE

The cable can provide sideways resistance that dumb-bells and barbells can't.

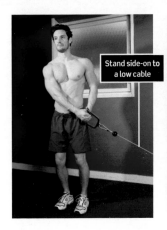

Stand side-on to a low cable

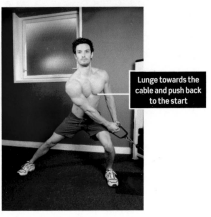

Lunge towards the cable and push back to the start

Bulgarian split squat

Target: quads, glutes

By placing one foot on a bench behind you, you deactivate that leg and transfer the emphasis to the front leg, giving you a unilateral workout.

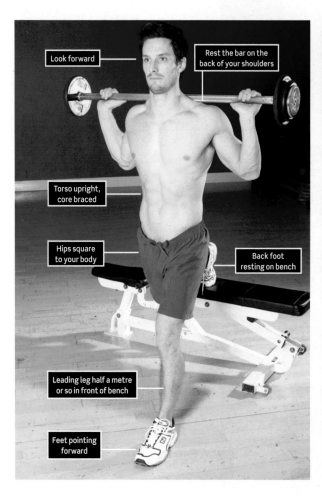

Look forward

Rest the bar on the back of your shoulders

Torso upright, core braced

Hips square to your body

Back foot resting on bench

Leading leg half a metre or so in front of bench

Feet pointing forward

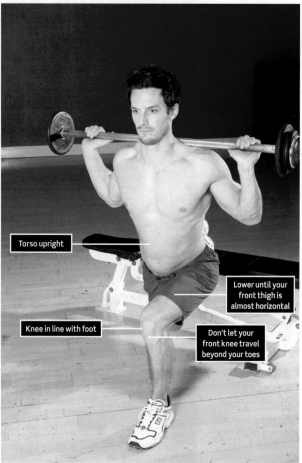

Torso upright

Lower until your front thigh is almost horizontal

Knee in line with foot

Don't let your front knee travel beyond your toes

Variations

DUMB-BELL BULGARIAN SPLIT SQUAT

Dumb-bells help to make the exercise easier but don't allow you to carry as much weight, so they're useful when learning this exercise.

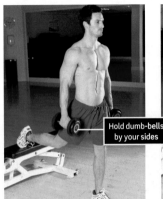
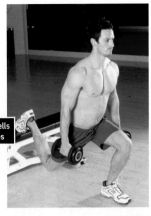

Hold dumb-bells by your sides

SWISS BALL BULGARIAN SPLIT SQUAT

With your back foot on a Swiss ball, the move becomes significantly more unstable, making your front leg work even harder.

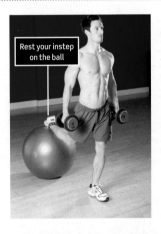
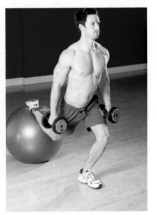

Rest your instep on the ball

SWISS BALL BULGARIAN SPLIT SQUAT WITH TWIST

Promote good balance and co-ordination with a move that works your body through several planes at the same time.

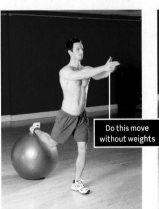
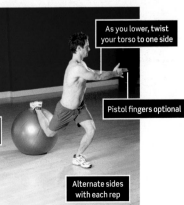

Do this move without weights

As you lower, twist your torso to one side

Pistol fingers optional

Alternate sides with each rep

Romanian deadlift

Target: hamstrings

The best way to build muscle mass on the backs of your thighs. Ensure perfect form to protect your lower back.

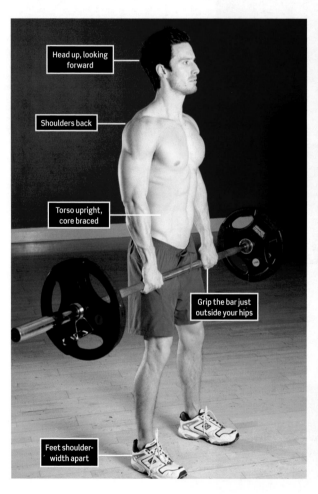

Head up, looking forward

Shoulders back

Torso upright, core braced

Grip the bar just outside your hips

Feet shoulder-width apart

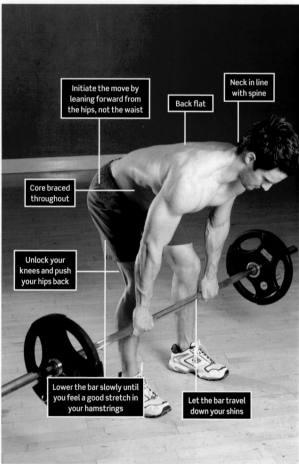

Initiate the move by leaning forward from the hips, not the waist

Back flat

Neck in line with spine

Core braced throughout

Unlock your knees and push your hips back

Lower the bar slowly until you feel a good stretch in your hamstrings

Let the bar travel down your shins

Variations

ONE-LEG ROMANIAN DEADLIFT

Work each leg independently and promote leg stability. A great way to warm up your hams for heavyweight Romanian deadlifts.

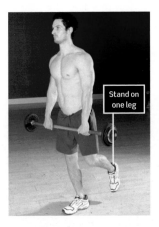

Stand on one leg

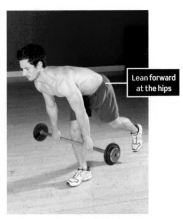

Lean forward at the hips

SPLIT DUMB-BELL ROMANIAN DEADLIFT

As well as working each leg independently, this move is highly functional as it replicates the standard way most people bend down to pick up items.

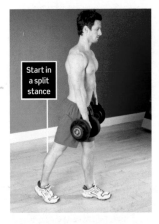

Start in a split stance

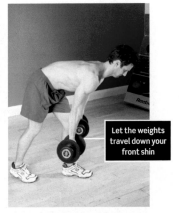

Let the weights travel down your front shin

STIFF-LEGGED ROMANIAN DEADLIFT

Keeping your legs straight places greater emphasis on your hamstrings but can put extra pressure on your lower back, so ensure perfect form, and build up the weight slowly.

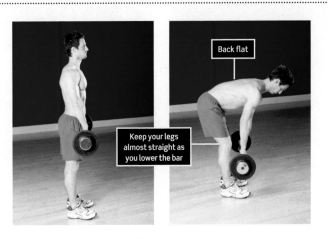

Back flat

Keep your legs almost straight as you lower the bar

Swiss ball leg curl

Target: hamstrings
Use your own bodyweight to target your hamstrings.

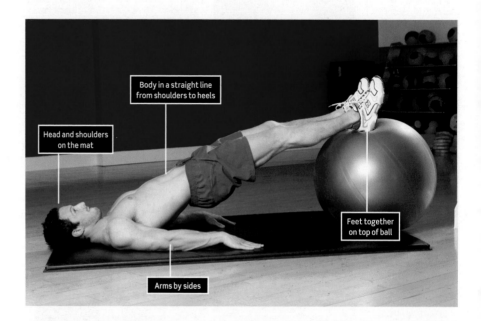

Body in a straight line from shoulders to heels

Head and shoulders on the mat

Feet together on top of ball

Arms by sides

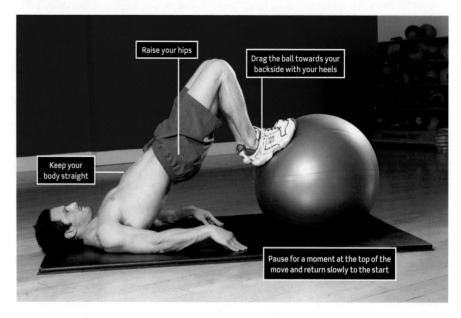

Raise your hips

Drag the ball towards your backside with your heels

Keep your body straight

Pause for a moment at the top of the move and return slowly to the start

Variations

ONE-LEG SWISS BALL LEG CURL

Each leg has to work twice as hard to stabilise your bodyweight on the wobbly ball.

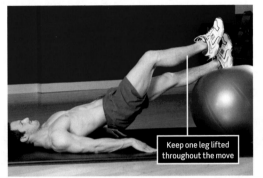

Keep one leg lifted throughout the move

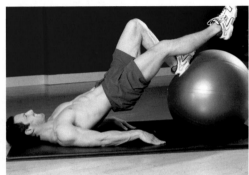

SWISS BALL HIP RAISE AND LEG CURL

A combination move that starts by exercising your hip flexors (tops of your thighs) and then moves on to target your hamstrings.

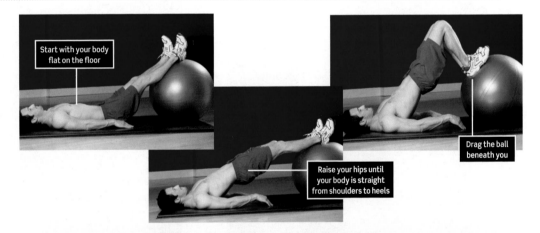

Start with your body flat on the floor

Raise your hips until your body is straight from shoulders to heels

Drag the ball beneath you

DOUBLE MEDICINE BALL LEG CURL

Two legs, two balls. Extra co-ordination is required to pull off this move, making your core work hard to keep your body straight.

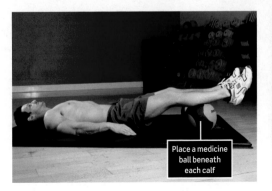

Place a medicine ball beneath each calf

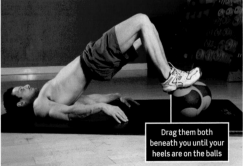

Drag them both beneath you until your heels are on the balls

Standing calf raise

Target: calves

Your calves are among the hardest muscles in the body to grow because they already work hard simply by walking around. Use heavy weights and low reps to force your calf muscles into growth.

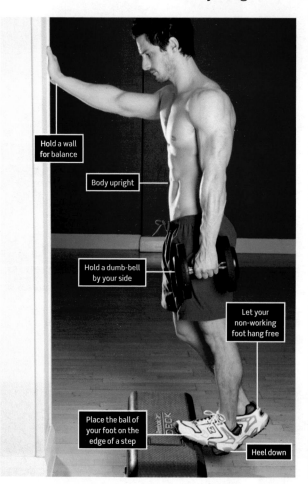

Hold a wall for balance

Body upright

Hold a dumb-bell by your side

Let your non-working foot hang free

Place the ball of your foot on the edge of a step

Heel down

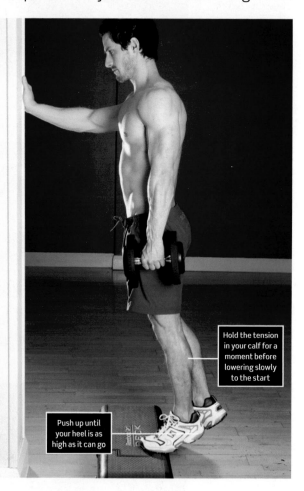

Hold the tension in your calf for a moment before lowering slowly to the start

Push up until your heel is as high as it can go

Variations

SEATED DUMB-BELL CALF RAISE

Hold a weight on your knees to provide resistance across the full range of motion.

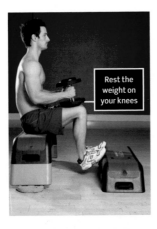

Rest the weight on your knees

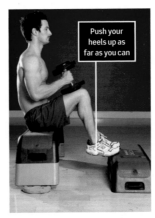

Push your heels up as far as you can

JUMPING CALF RAISE

Explosive moves like this target your fast-twitch muscle fibres that have the most potential for growth.

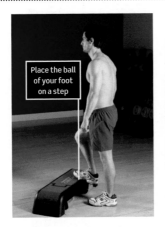

Place the ball of your foot on a step

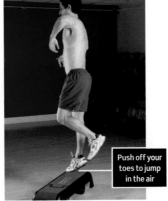

Push off your toes to jump in the air

SUPINE SWISS BALL CALF RAISE

Your calves are forced to stabilise your entire body, making them more efficient when it comes to lifting weight.

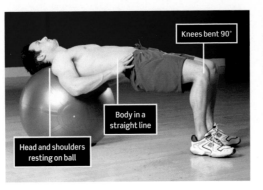

Knees bent 90°

Body in a straight line

Head and shoulders resting on ball

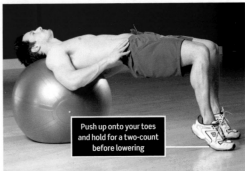

Push up onto your toes and hold for a two-count before lowering

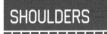

SHOULDERS

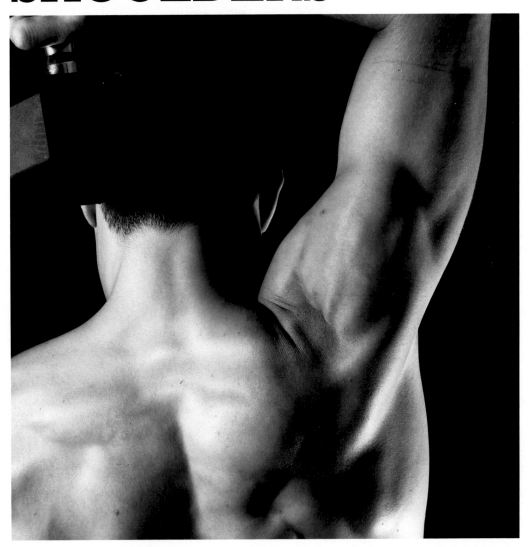

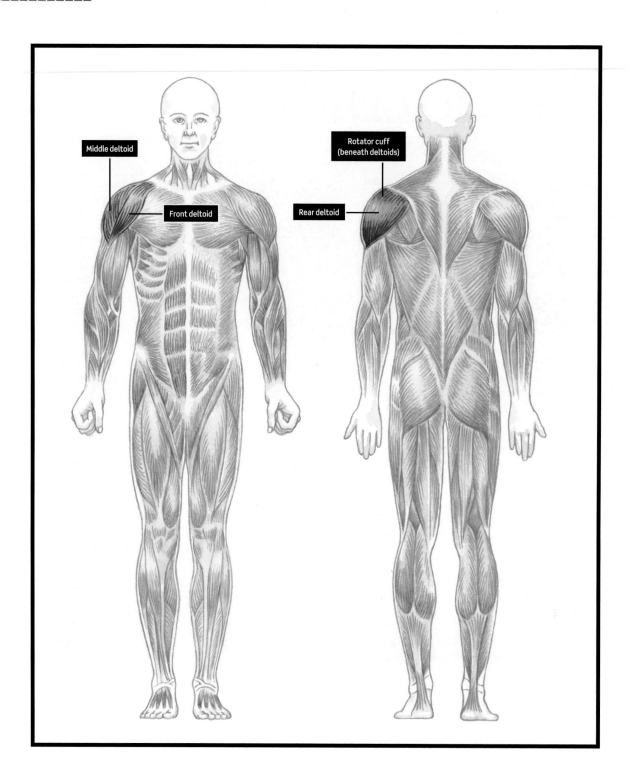

Middle deltoid

Front deltoid

Rotator cuff (beneath deltoids)

Rear deltoid

SHOULDERS

The shoulder is one of the most complex joints in your body. A ball of bone at the top of your upper-arm bone (humerus) sits in a scoop of bone on your shoulder blade, allowing your arm to move in numerous directions. Moving your arm up, down, out and back involves a large number of muscles, including the pecs on your chest, the lats and traps on your back, and the deltoids on the shoulder joint. And it's the deltoids we'll be focusing on in this section.

Your delts come in three parts: front, middle and rear (or anterior, medial and posterior if you want to sound more intelligent). It's important to target all parts of your deltoids or you can end up with muscle imbalances that lead to injury. For example, if you do lots of bench pressing, but no rowing movements, your front delts will become stronger than your rear delts, which will restrict the range of movement your shoulder joint can achieve, which in turn will lead to you yelping in pain after some kid asks, 'Hey mister, can you can you throw my ball back?'

Assisting the big muscles that manipulate the shoulder are smaller, internal muscles collectively known as your rotator cuff. These muscles aren't very glamorous – they won't grow large and impressive – but they are vital for preventing injury to a very delicate joint. These muscles stabilise the shoulder joint and allow you to rotate your arms as well as lift them (imagine the action of throwing a ball). If these small muscles aren't given sufficient attention in the gym, they will fail to support the larger muscles such as the deltoids when you train them, which can lead to niggling injuries.

Before any heavy shoulder exercises, doing rotator cuff exercises such as internal and external rotations (p148) will help to warm up your entire shoulder girdle and prepare you for the heavy lifts to follow.

Main exercises

Shoulder press — 136

Seated dumb-bell shoulder press — 138

Alternating dumb-bell shoulder press — 140

Lateral raise — 142

Lying reverse lateral raise — 144

Cuban press — 146

Internal dumb-bell rotation — 148

Shoulder press

Target: deltoids

Add size and strength to your shoulders
with th must-do exercise.

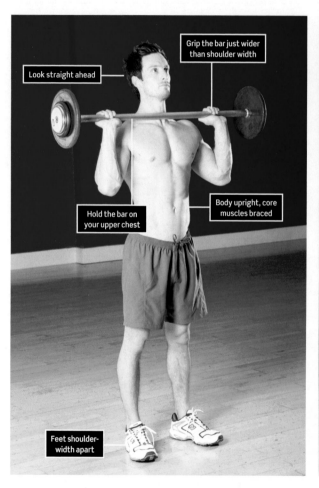

Look straight ahead

Grip the bar just wider
than shoulder width

Hold the bar on
your upper chest

Body upright, core
muscles braced

Feet shoulder-
width apart

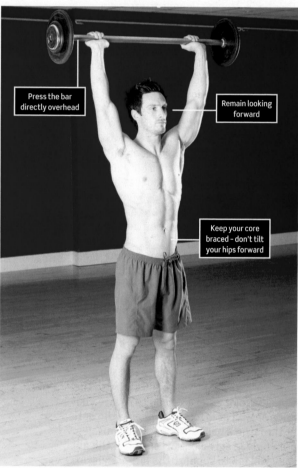

Press the bar
directly overhead

Remain looking
forward

Keep your core
braced – don't tilt
your hips forward

Variations

PUSH PRESS

Use the power in your legs to initiate the move. This can help you lift more weight and prevent you from leaning back at the start of the move.

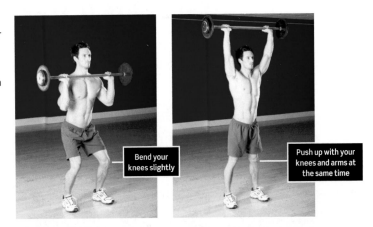

Bend your knees slightly

Push up with your knees and arms at the same time

INVERTED SHOULDER PRESS

Got no weights? This is the easiest way to train your shoulders using your own bodyweight.

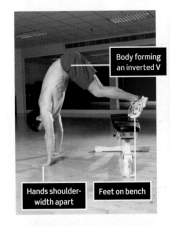

Body forming an inverted V

Hands shoulder-width apart

Feet on bench

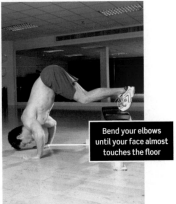

Bend your elbows until your face almost touches the floor

SHOULDER PRESS WITH ROTATION

Work your shoulders and core at the same time, using the muscles of your midsection to control the rotation.

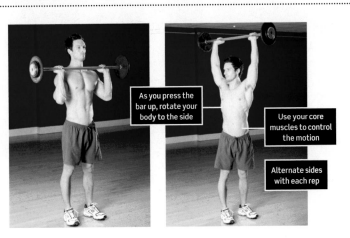

As you press the bar up, rotate your body to the side

Use your core muscles to control the motion

Alternate sides with each rep

Seated dumb-bell shoulder press

Target: **deltoids**

Using dumb-bells means you don't have to worry about your head getting in the way of the bar, your hands move in a more natural arc, and you train each shoulder independently.

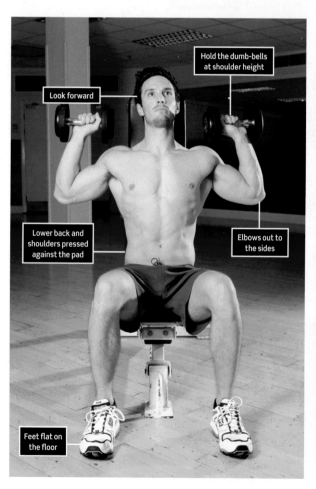

Look forward

Hold the dumb-bells at shoulder height

Lower back and shoulders pressed against the pad

Elbows out to the sides

Feet flat on the floor

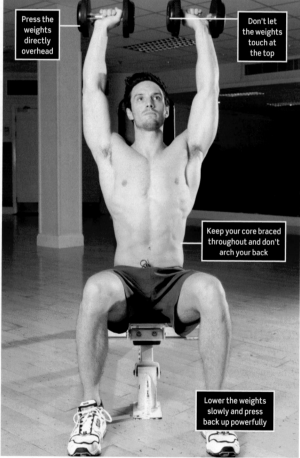

Press the weights directly overhead

Don't let the weights touch at the top

Keep your core braced throughout and don't arch your back

Lower the weights slowly and press back up powerfully

Variations

HAMMER GRIP SEATED DUMB-BELL SHOULDER PRESS

Those with poor shoulder flexibility will find this grip easier, and it draws your elbows forward, which recruits your chest muscles to help with the move.

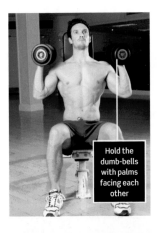
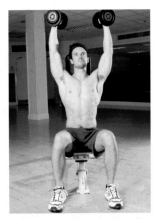

Hold the dumb-bells with palms facing each other

SWISS BALL SEATED DUMB-BELL SHOULDER PRESS

Give your core stabilising muscles a workout along with your shoulders by keeping your torso steady during the move.

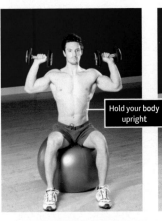
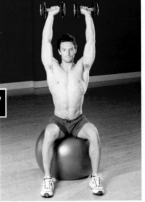

Hold your body upright

ARNOLD PRESS

This combines a pressing motion with a rotational one, hitting your delts from several angles in a single move.

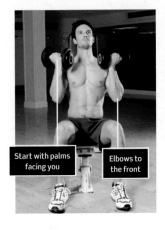
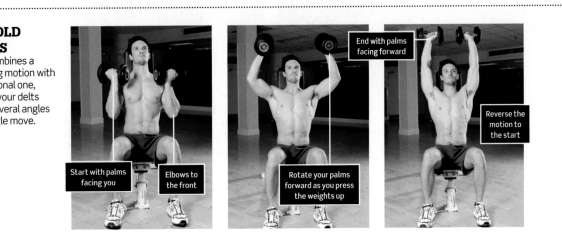

Start with palms facing you

Elbows to the front

Rotate your palms forward as you press the weights up

End with palms facing forward

Reverse the motion to the start

Alternating dumb-bell shoulder press

Target: **deltoids**

Focus on one side of your body at a time to make each shoulder work as hard as possible.

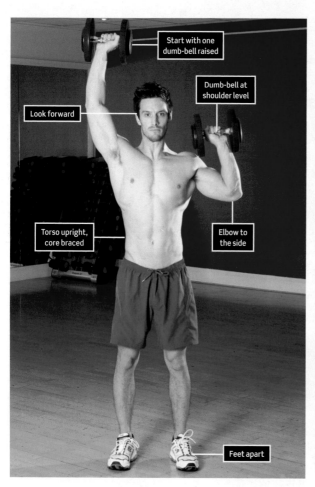

Start with one dumb-bell raised

Dumb-bell at shoulder level

Look forward

Torso upright, core braced

Elbow to the side

Feet apart

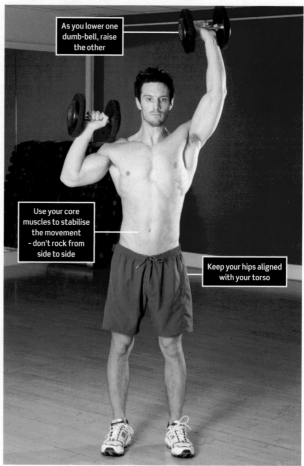

As you lower one dumb-bell, raise the other

Use your core muscles to stabilise the movement – don't rock from side to side

Keep your hips aligned with your torso

Variations

ROTATING SQUAT PRESS

This turns a shoulder move into a whole-body move, working your legs, back, shoulders, arms and core all at the same time.

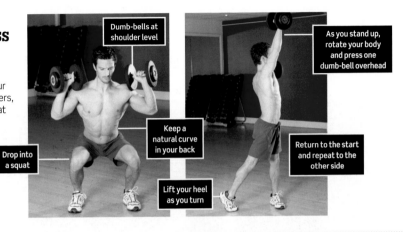

Dumb-bells at shoulder level

As you stand up, rotate your body and press one dumb-bell overhead

Keep a natural curve in your back

Drop into a squat

Return to the start and repeat to the other side

Lift your heel as you turn

ALTERNATING WIDE-SHOULDER PRESS

Hit your delts from a new angle with this variation on a classic move.

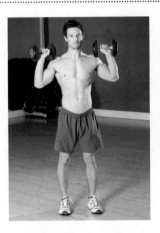
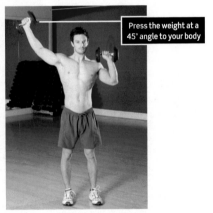

Press the weight at a 45° angle to your body

CABLE SPLIT SQUAT TO OVERHEAD PRESS

A whole-body move that uses a cable to maintain a constant resistance on your shoulders.

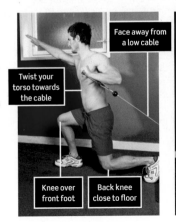

Face away from a low cable

Twist your torso towards the cable

Knee over front foot

Back knee close to floor

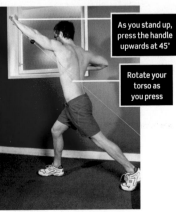

As you stand up, press the handle upwards at 45°

Rotate your torso as you press

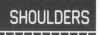

Lateral raise

Target: **middle deltoid**

Keep the weight light and isolate your middle shoulders with this single-joint move.

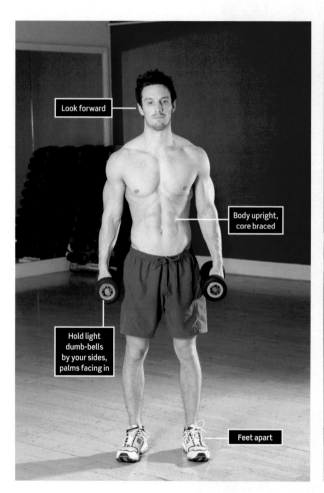

Look forward

Body upright, core braced

Hold light dumb-bells by your sides, palms facing in

Feet apart

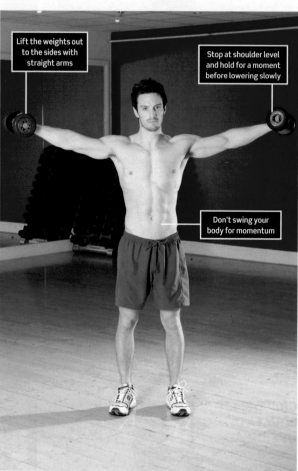

Lift the weights out to the sides with straight arms

Stop at shoulder level and hold for a moment before lowering slowly

Don't swing your body for momentum

Variations

FRONT RAISE
Transfer the emphasis to your front shoulders.

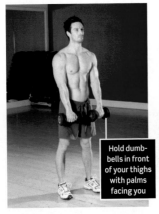

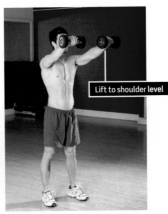

Lift to shoulder level

Hold dumb-bells in front of your thighs with palms facing you

FRONT/ LATERAL RAISE
Alternating sides each time works both the front and middle shoulders.

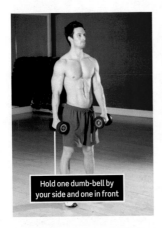

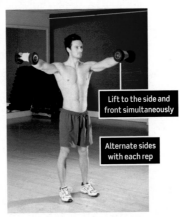

Lift to the side and front simultaneously

Alternate sides with each rep

Hold one dumb-bell by your side and one in front

CABLE SQUAT TO OVERHEAD RAISE
Work your front, middle and rear shoulders, as well as your legs, back and core with this compound movement.

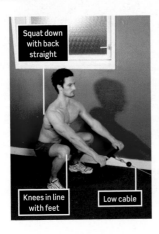

Squat down with back straight

Knees in line with feet

Low cable

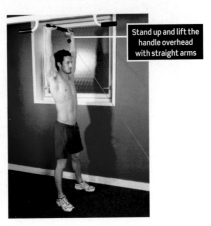

Stand up and lift the handle overhead with straight arms

Lying reverse lateral raise

Target: **rear deltoid**

Target those hard-to-reach rear shoulders, and give your upper-back muscles a workout into the bargain.

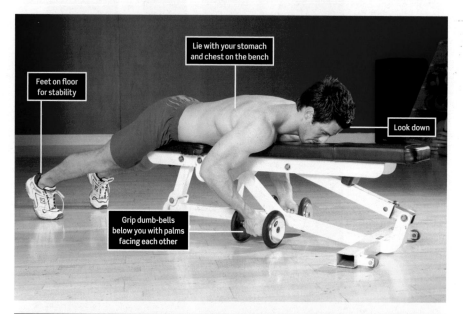

Feet on floor for stability

Lie with your stomach and chest on the bench

Look down

Grip dumb-bells below you with palms facing each other

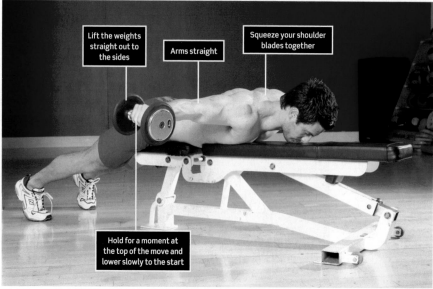

Lift the weights straight out to the sides

Arms straight

Squeeze your shoulder blades together

Hold for a moment at the top of the move and lower slowly to the start

Variations

HIGH CABLE WIDE PULL

Using a high, wide bar keeps the emphasis on your rear shoulders rather than your back.

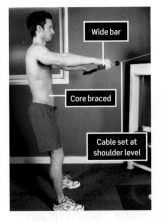

Wide bar

Core braced

Cable set at shoulder level

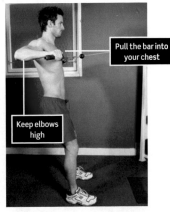

Pull the bar into your chest

Keep elbows high

DIAGONAL CABLE RAISE

The pressure starts on your front delts and transfers to your rear delts as you raise the cable.

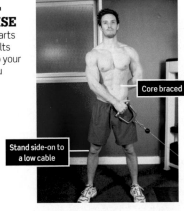

Core braced

Stand side-on to a low cable

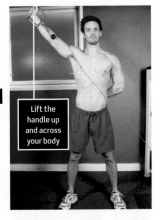

Lift the handle up and across your body

HIGH CABLE REVERSE FLYE

The flye motion stops your arms from doing any of the work and places the tension on your rear shoulders and back.

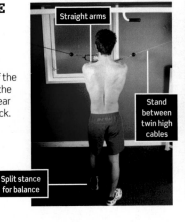

Straight arms

Stand between twin high cables

Split stance for balance

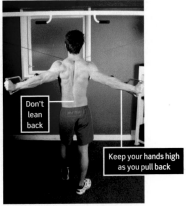

Don't lean back

Keep your hands high as you pull back

Cuban press

Target: rotator cuff

This move works the smaller, internal muscles of the shoulder that control the rotational movement of the shoulder joint. A strong rotator cuff will prevent injuries from heavy lifting.

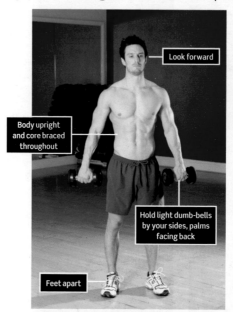

Look forward

Body upright and core braced throughout

Hold light dumb-bells by your sides, palms facing back

Feet apart

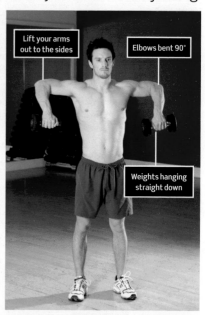

Lift your arms out to the sides

Elbows bent 90°

Weights hanging straight down

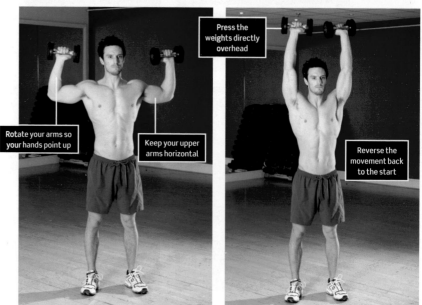

Rotate your arms so your hands point up

Keep your upper arms horizontal

Press the weights directly overhead

Reverse the movement back to the start

Variations

LYING CUBAN PRESS

A change of angle places your rotator cuff muscles under different stresses.

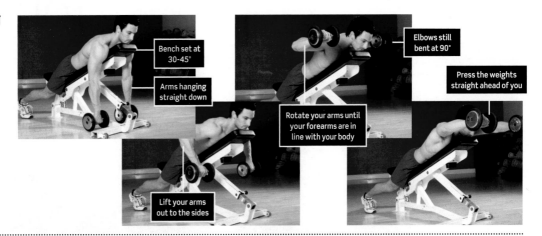

Bench set at 30-45°

Arms hanging straight down

Lift your arms out to the sides

Rotate your arms until your forearms are in line with your body

Elbows still bent at 90°

Press the weights straight ahead of you

SWISS BALL LYING CUBAN PRESS

Keeping the ball steady helps to ensure that your posture is correct while you perform the move.

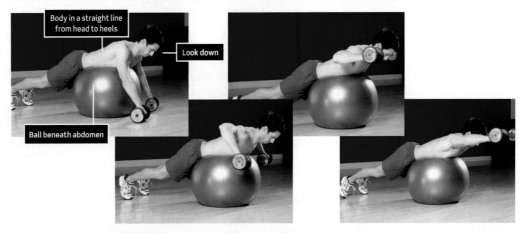

Body in a straight line from head to heels

Look down

Ball beneath abdomen

STANDING FOUR-POINT PRESS

Combine pressing and rotating the shoulders in one move – don't overdo the weights while performing this.

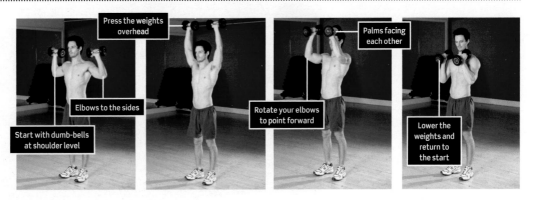

Press the weights overhead

Elbows to the sides

Start with dumb-bells at shoulder level

Rotate your elbows to point forward

Palms facing each other

Lower the weights and return to the start

Internal dumb-bell rotation

Target: **rotator cuff**

This move is a must-do as a warm-up before any shoulder workout to help prevent injuries.

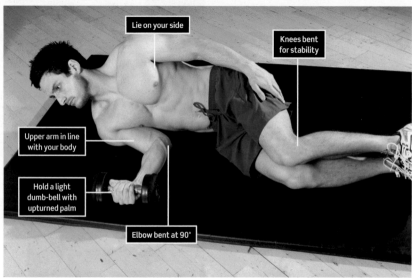

Lie on your side

Knees bent for stability

Upper arm in line with your body

Hold a light dumb-bell with upturned palm

Elbow bent at 90°

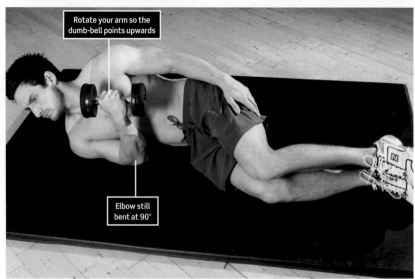

Rotate your arm so the dumb-bell points upwards

Elbow still bent at 90°

Variations

EXTERNAL DUMB-BELL ROTATION

Move your shoulder in the opposite direction to the internal rotation.

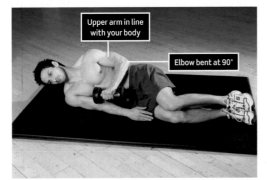

Upper arm in line with your body

Elbow bent at 90°

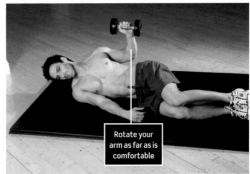

Rotate your arm as far as is comfortable

INTERNAL CABLE ROTATION

The cable places slightly different forces on the shoulder muscles compared with dumb-bells.

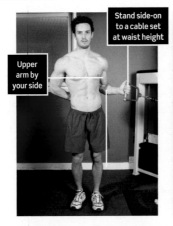

Stand side-on to a cable set at waist height

Upper arm by your side

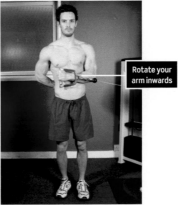

Rotate your arm inwards

EXTERNAL CABLE ROTATION

Twist your arm outwards instead of inwards.

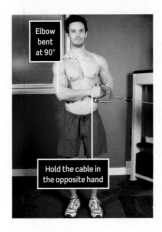

Elbow bent at 90°

Hold the cable in the opposite hand

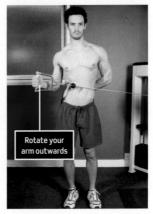

Rotate your arm outwards

TOTAL BODY

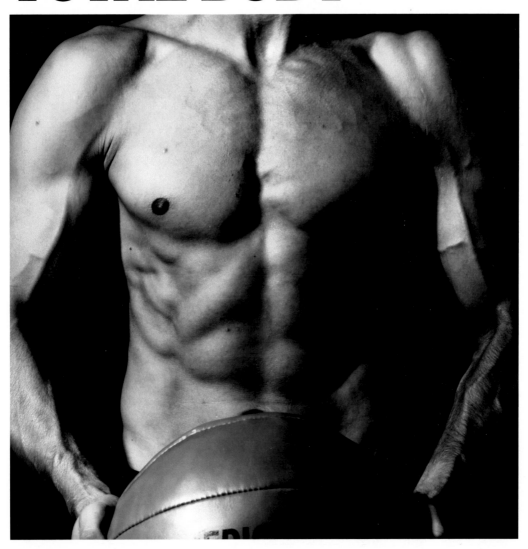

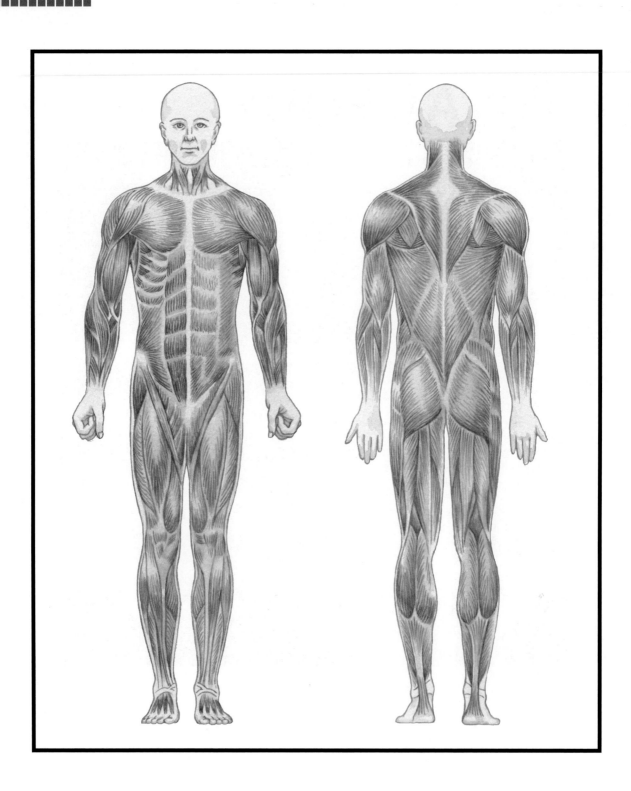

TOTAL BODY

Some exercises work so many muscles that they can't be categorised by body parts, which is why they get a chapter all of their own.

These exercises are either compound movements or combination moves. Compound exercises are when a single action requires the body to move several joints at once, and as a result you have to work many different muscle groups at the same time. For example a deadlift (p154) seems like a fairly simple action – you're just picking something up from the floor – yet it requires you to move at the ankles, knees and hips simultaneously, while supporting the weight with your shoulders and stabilising your spine as you raise the bar. This simple action works all the muscles of your legs, your back and shoulders, your core muscles and your forearm muscles, which are required to grip the bar. It's a whole-body workout in a single move.

Other exercises in this section take the idea of compound movements further by introducing dynamic elements. The hang clean (p156), for example, requires you to hoist a barbell up in front of you powerfully enough to be able to flip it onto your front shoulders. Not only does this use a lot of different muscles, but the explosive movement required to raise the bar at speed fires up your fast-twitch muscle fibres – the ones involved in dynamic movements – which have the most potential for growth. (Slow-twitch fibres are the ones made for endurance, and have less growth potential. That's why distance runners tend to be skinnier than sprinters.)

Combination exercises are when you stitch together two or more moves to create a new exercise. We've given four examples on p160-161, but you are only limited by your imagination when it comes to creating new combo exercises. Grab a pair of dumb-bells and there's no reason why you can't perform a squat-to-clean-to-press-to-lunge-to-curl-to-deadlift-to-row combo. By linking exercises like this you keep your work rate high, which is great for burning fat, saving time and training your body to function as a single unit.

Main exercises

Deadlift	154
Hang clean	156
Woodchop	158
Lunge to press	160

Deadlift

Target: **quads, glutes, hamstrings, back, core**

The deadlift works your lower and upper body at the same time in one mass-building compound move. Keep your core muscles tight to avoid lower-back pain.

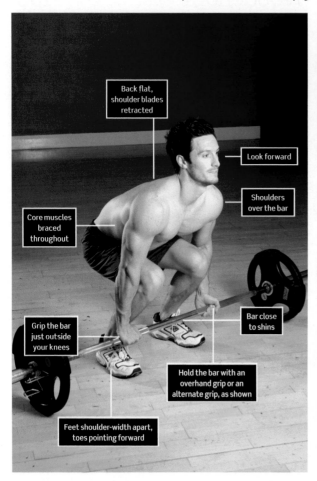

Back flat, shoulder blades retracted

Look forward

Shoulders over the bar

Core muscles braced throughout

Grip the bar just outside your knees

Bar close to shins

Hold the bar with an overhand grip or an alternate grip, as shown

Feet shoulder-width apart, toes pointing forward

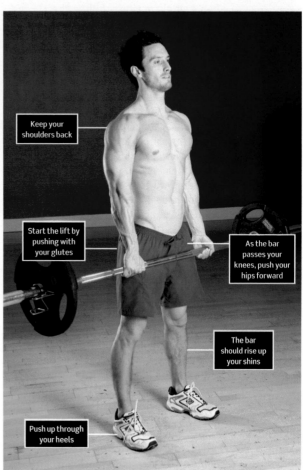

Keep your shoulders back

Start the lift by pushing with your glutes

As the bar passes your knees, push your hips forward

The bar should rise up your shins

Push up through your heels

Variations

SNATCH-GRIP DEADLIFT

Hold the bar with a wider grip to place greater emphasis on your upper-back (trapezius) muscles.

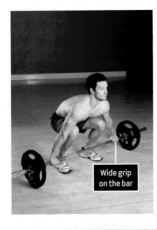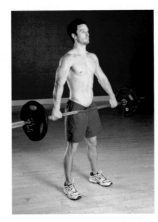

Wide grip on the bar

REDUCED DEADLIFT

If you find the range of motion of normal deadlifts too strenuous – especially if you already have lower-back problems – start with the weights raised on blocks.

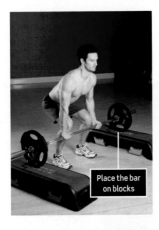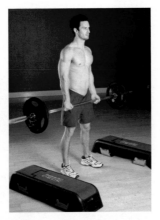

Place the bar on blocks

INCREASED DEADLIFT

To increase your range of motion and improve your ability to lift the bar off the floor, try this exaggerated deadlift – just keep the weights light to begin with.

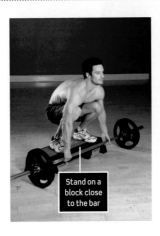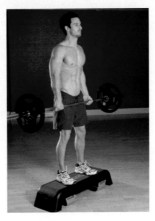

Stand on a block close to the bar

Hang clean

Target: **hamstrings, glutes, calves, back, shoulders**
This exercise works your body from top to toe in a dynamic, powerful movement.

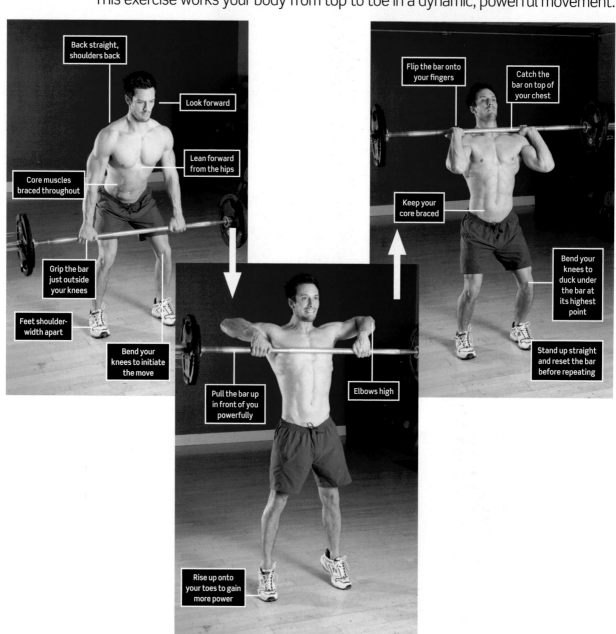

Back straight, shoulders back

Look forward

Lean forward from the hips

Core muscles braced throughout

Grip the bar just outside your knees

Feet shoulder-width apart

Bend your knees to initiate the move

Flip the bar onto your fingers

Catch the bar on top of your chest

Keep your core braced

Bend your knees to duck under the bar at its highest point

Stand up straight and reset the bar before repeating

Pull the bar up in front of you powerfully

Elbows high

Rise up onto your toes to gain more power

Variations

SNATCH

Duck under the bar to 'catch' it overhead. This requires excellent co-ordination and shoulder flexibility, so try it with a light bar to begin with.

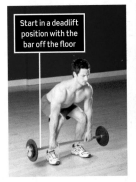
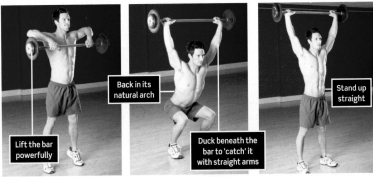

Start in a deadlift position with the bar off the floor

Lift the bar powerfully

Back in its natural arch

Duck beneath the bar to 'catch' it with straight arms

Stand up straight

ONE-ARM DUMB-BELL SNATCH

Work each side of your body independently – especially useful for sports conditioning.

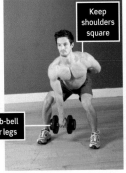
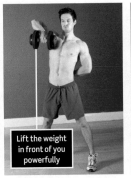
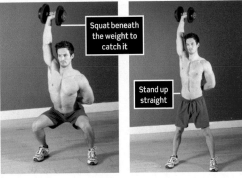

Keep shoulders square

Hold one dumb-bell between your legs

Lift the weight in front of you powerfully

Squat beneath the weight to catch it

Stand up straight

CLEAN AND JERK

This exercise targets so many muscle groups it's a workout in itself. Ensure perfect form throughout.

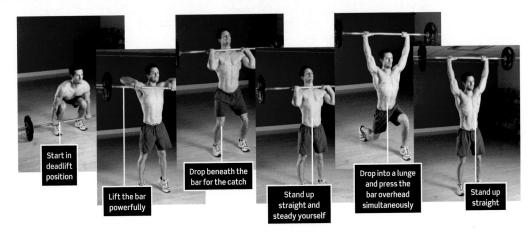

Start in deadlift position

Lift the bar powerfully

Drop beneath the bar for the catch

Stand up straight and steady yourself

Drop into a lunge and press the bar overhead simultaneously

Stand up straight

Woodchop

Target: **abdominals, lower back, quads, shoulders**
This rotational lift builds the connection between your upper and lower body and creates a strong core for sports.

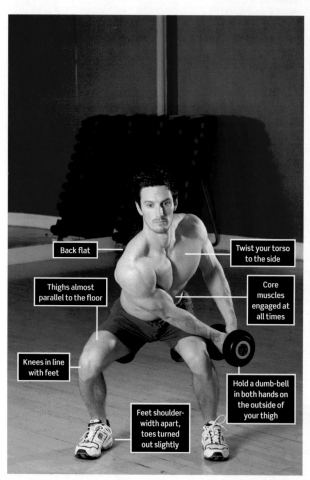

Back flat

Thighs almost parallel to the floor

Knees in line with feet

Twist your torso to the side

Core muscles engaged at all times

Hold a dumb-bell in both hands on the outside of your thigh

Feet shoulder-width apart, toes turned out slightly

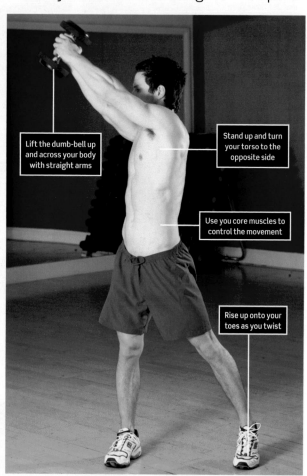

Lift the dumb-bell up and across your body with straight arms

Stand up and turn your torso to the opposite side

Use you core muscles to control the movement

Rise up onto your toes as you twist

Variations

CABLE WOODCHOP

Work your body in the opposing plane to the standard dumb-bell woodchop.

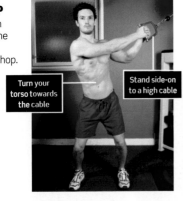

Turn your torso towards the cable

Stand side-on to a high cable

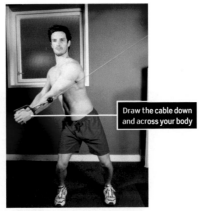

Draw the cable down and across your body

CABLE LOW-TO-HIGH WOODCHOP

The cable provides constant resistance across the full range of the exercise.

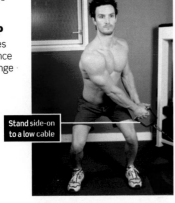

Stand side-on to a low cable

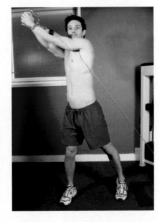

WOODCHOP LUNGE

The woodchop/lunge combination requires your body to work horizontally, vertically and rotationally at the same time. It's a great way to build co-ordination and functional strength.

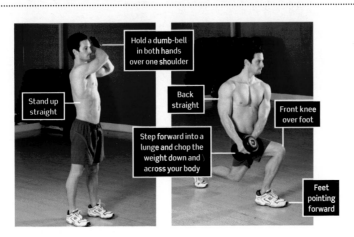

Hold a dumb-bell in both hands over one shoulder

Stand up straight

Back straight

Front knee over foot

Step forward into a lunge and chop the weight down and across your body

Feet pointing forward

Lunge to press

Target: **quads, glutes, hamstrings, shoulders, triceps**

All these exercises combine upper- and lower-body moves to get twice the workout in half the time.

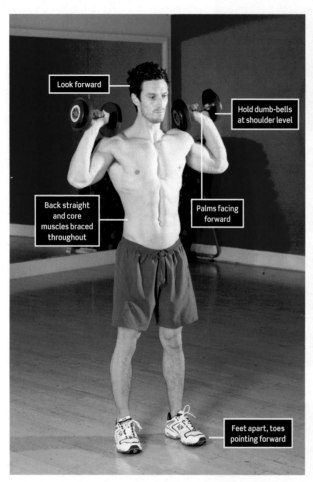

Look forward

Hold dumb-bells at shoulder level

Back straight and core muscles braced throughout

Palms facing forward

Feet apart, toes pointing forward

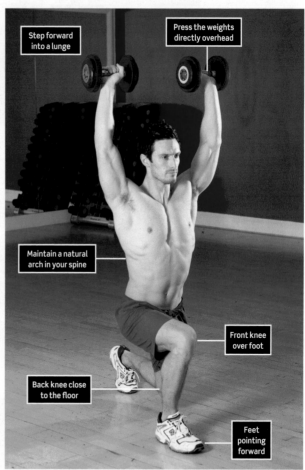

Step forward into a lunge

Press the weights directly overhead

Maintain a natural arch in your spine

Front knee over foot

Back knee close to the floor

Feet pointing forward

Variations

SQUAT TO CURL TO PRESS

Combine three separate exercise to get your body working as a single unit.

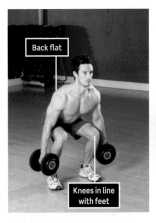

Back flat

Knees in line with feet

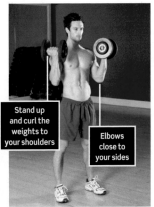

Stand up and curl the weights to your shoulders

Elbows close to your sides

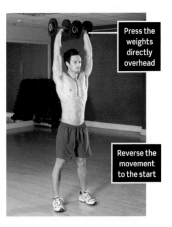

Press the weights directly overhead

Reverse the movement to the start

ROMANIAN DEADLIFT TO ROW

Work your back and hamstring muscles together with this classic combo.

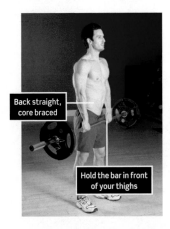

Back straight, core braced

Hold the bar in front of your thighs

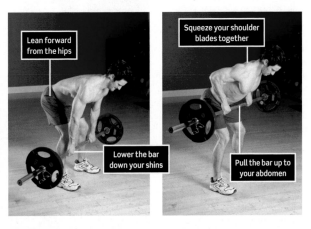

Lean forward from the hips

Lower the bar down your shins

Squeeze your shoulder blades together

Pull the bar up to your abdomen

SWISS BALL JACKNIFE TO PRESS-UP

This combination move targets your abs, hips, chest and triceps.

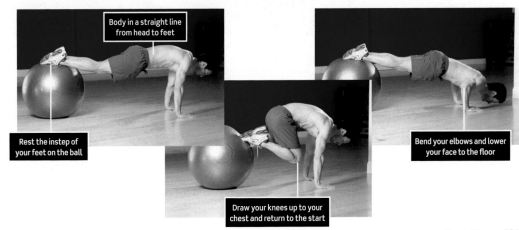

Body in a straight line from head to feet

Rest the instep of your feet on the ball

Draw your knees up to your chest and return to the start

Bend your elbows and lower your face to the floor

Stretch it out

After every workout stretch your muscles to ease recovery and reduce injuries

Stretching is a subject that causes a great deal of disagreement among weight-training experts. There have been studies that suggest stretching offers no obvious improvement in performance and doesn't prevent injuries, and therefore you shouldn't bother with it. Some trainers will recommend static stretches before a workout, while others insist that they should only be used afterwards.

At *Men's Fitness* magazine we take a fairly traditional approach to stretching based on our own experience. We advocate dynamic stretching before a workout (see p12 for your pre-workout routine) and static stretching once you have completed your workout and warmed down sufficiently.

WHY STRETCH?
When you perform a static stretch, you relax a muscle and hold it under tension for a specific period of time without moving. This helps to lengthen the muscle after it has contracted as a result of weight training and provides a range of benefits:

• **Greater flexibility** – stretching will allow you to perform exercises across a wider range of movement, improving your muscle-building effect.

• **Fewer injuries** – when you have less tension in your muscles you significantly reduce your chances of tearing muscle fibres or tendons when you perform dynamic movements.

• **Faster recovery** – stretching improves blood flow to your muscles and helps to flush out toxins, meaning you'll be ready for your next workout sooner.

• **Better posture** – tense muscles can pull your shoulders, hips and spine out of

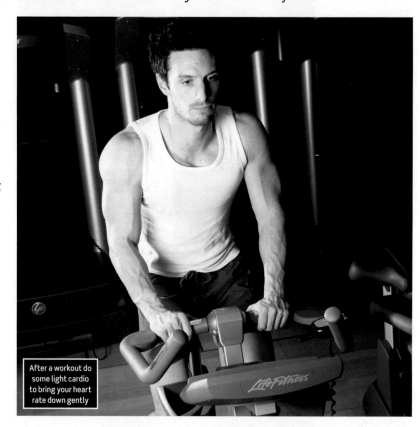

After a workout do some light cardio to bring your heart rate down gently

alignment, which can cause back pain, not to mention making you stoop – and that's never a good look.

HOW TO STRETCH
After you've finished your workout, spend five to ten minutes doing some gentle cardio, such as cycling on an exercise bike, to bring your heart rate back to normal gradually. Then perform the stretches demonstrated opposite, paying particular attention to any muscle

groups that you have targeted during your workout.

Get into the stretch position and allow your muscle to relax. As you place pressure on the muscle you should be able to feel it relaxing and lengthening. You can slowly increase the pressure on the muscle throughout the duration of the stretch, but never force it or 'bounce' it, or you could end up damaging the muscle. If you feel pain, stop immediately. Hold each stretch for 15-30 seconds.

CALVES

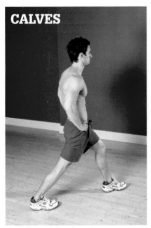

Press your back heel down to feel the stretch in your rear calf.

HAMSTRINGS

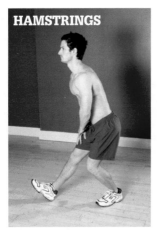

Lean forward gently to feel the stretch in the hamstring of your front leg.

QUADS

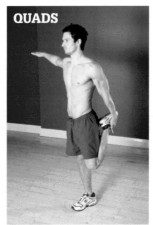

Hold your foot and push your hips forward to feel the stretch in your thigh.

HIP FLEXORS

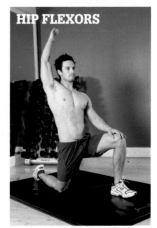

Keep your body upright and push your hips forward.

ADDUCTORS

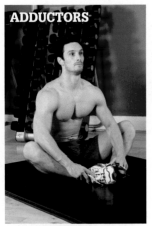

Touch your soles together and press gently on your knees with your elbows.

GLUTES

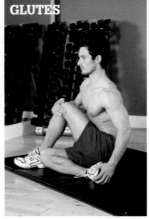

Sit upright and pull gently on your knee to feel the stretch in your buttock.

ABS

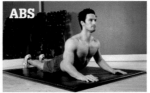

Raise your shoulders without stressing your lower back.

LATS

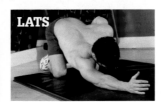

Press down on your arm to feel the stretch down your sides.

LOWER BACK

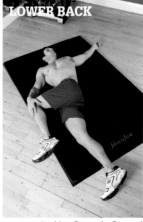

Keep your shoulders flat on the floor and press your knee down.

CHEST

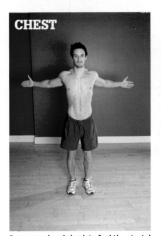

Press your hands back to feel the stretch across your chest.

TRAPS

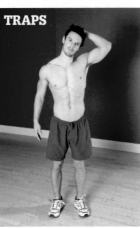

Pull gently on your head and push your opposite shoulder down.

TRICEPS

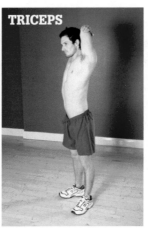

Point your fingers down your back and pull gently on your elbow with your other hand.

BICEPS

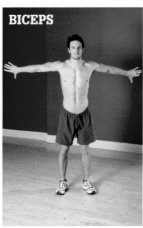

Point your thumbs down and press your arms behind you.

How to build a workout

You've seen the exercises, now here's how to combine them into an effective workout routine

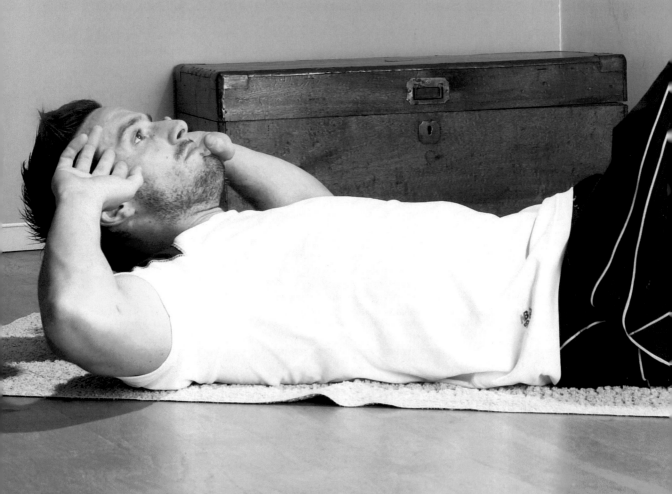

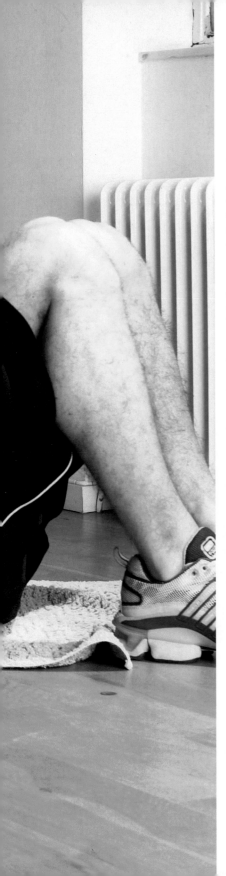

When you go to a gym, or even if you train from home, it's vital to have a clear idea in your mind of what you want to achieve from your workout. Then you can select the exercises that will best help you to achieve your goals.

The first thing you need to realise is that there is no such thing as the perfect workout – a single routine that you can perform again and again to help you build muscle and burn fat. The human body has more than 650 muscles and you can't hope to work all of them thoroughly in one single workout. You have to keep changing and developing your training regime because different exercises will affect your muscles in different ways. If you always stick to the same few exercises your body will soon adapt to the stresses placed on it and stop responding. In short, doing the same workout time and time again won't give you the body you want.

For that reason we haven't provided you with a specific workout plan to follow in this book, but we will give you the tools to create your own workouts. Firstly, we've given you more than 240 exercises for you to choose from. Now we'll provide you with the knowledge you need to help structure your workouts, and over the next few pages we'll give you examples of workouts that you can use as templates for your own gym sessions.

THINGS TO THINK ABOUT WHEN PLANNING A WORKOUT

1 What exercises should you do?
That depends on what you want to achieve. It might be that you want to add muscle mass to a specific part of your body. Or perhaps you want to burn off fat to look more defined. You could be training for a sport or trying to build core stability to improve posture and athletic performance. Your goals will affect the structure of your workout – the exercises you do, the sets and reps you choose, the rest periods you take and the weights you select. You can find out more about how to pick exercises to suit your goals in the examples on pages 166 to 173.

2 How many repetitions (reps) should you do?
When it comes to building muscle not all men are created equal. Different bodies will react differently to the same exercises, but there are a few general rules about sets and reps you can follow until you work out what works best for you. Low reps in the 4-8 range are considered best for building strength; reps in the 8-12 range are best for adding muscle mass; and high reps in the 15-25 range are best for muscle endurance.

In each case, for the set to be effective you need to be hitting 'failure' – the point at which you cannot complete another rep without breaking good form (not the point at which you can't move the weight at all) – at or around the specified rep range. If you get to 12 reps and feel you could do lots more then you are using a weight that's too light for you.

3 How many sets?
Once you've completed the specified number of reps of an exercise, you've finished one set. However your muscles can usually cope with extra work after a short rest, and the more work they do the more they will grow. So two to three sets is the norm for most exercises.

When you first start training you might want to do one set only until your muscles have become accustomed to training, then you can start to increase the sets you do after a few weeks. You'll need to use your own discretion to decide how many sets suits you, but your target muscle should feel fully exhausted by the time you finish the last set.

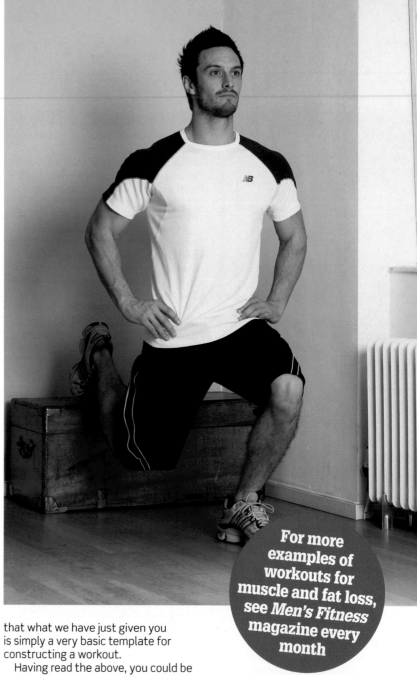

4 What about rest times?
The longer you rest between sets the more time you give your muscles to recover. If you are training for strength with low reps and heavy weights, you might want to rest for several minutes between sets to give your muscles the best chance of lifting the most weight. On the other hand, if you are training for endurance or fat loss, you might want to leave no rest time at all between sets to keep your work rate high and introduce a cardiovascular element to your workout.

Generally, the less time you spend between sets the better as this forces your muscles to work harder and stops you wasting time in the gym. Between 45 and 90 seconds is standard for muscle-building sets of 10-12 reps.

5 How many exercises per workout?
How much time do you have in the gym? If you are focusing on a particular body part, you can get away with doing fewer exercises, say four or five, and concentrate on the intensity. If you are hoping to do a full-body workout then you may need to do eight or more exercises to ensure that you hit all the areas you want to build.

6 How much time in the gym?
Longer does not always mean better in weight training. Various studies have suggested that after around 45 minutes of exercise you can actually start breaking down your muscle mass as your body begins to eat it up for fuel. There's no reason to spend two hours in the gym, and many men who do often spend it sitting around admiring themselves in the mirror. An hour, including warm-up, warm down and stretching, is as long as you need for an effective workout. Just use the time effectively.

NOW IGNORE ALL THE ABOVE
We're not suggesting you ignore it altogether, but you should understand that what we have just given you is simply a very basic template for constructing a workout.

Having read the above, you could be tempted to think that every workout should last at least one hour, include eight exercises, three sets of each, 10-12 reps per set, with 45 seconds rest between sets. Admittedly that's not a bad way to get started, but muscles love variety so you have to be prepared to rip up the rule book and vary your workouts regularly. Even something minor, such as changing the rep range or changing the rest time, can stimulate your muscles into new growth.

Over the next few pages you'll find some examples of workouts and how they achieve results. Use them to construct your own workouts, but be sure to make changes every few weeks to keep your muscles growing.

For more examples of workouts for muscle and fat loss, see *Men's Fitness* magazine every month

Sample Workout 1

Full-body workout

If you want to add muscle mass, then the full-body workout gives you the advantage that you can work a large number of muscle fibres in a limited time. Your body will respond by releasing a wave of hormones that will get to work making your muscles bigger and stronger.

The disadvantage of the full-body workout is that it is hard to fully exhaust all your muscles in the time available, so it makes sense to mix up your workouts with more muscle-specific sessions at other times (see the muscle-focus workout overleaf).

If you are new to training, the full-body workout is the best way to begin because you can get your muscles used to training without over-stressing any of them. Start by using light weights until you are confident that you have perfected the moves, then build up the weight over time.

ARRANGING YOUR WORKOUT
The key to full-body workouts is balance. For every pushing motion you should do a pulling one, and spend as much time on your lower body as upper. It's best to stick to compound exercises (multi-joint moves that work several muscle groups at once) as these will give the maximum muscle-building benefits in the time you have.

Be sure to leave any abs-specific exercises, such as crunches, to the end of your workout because you don't want to exhaust your core muscles before they're needed to stabilise your spine in big moves such as squats and rows. And make the first set of every exercise a light one to warm up your muscles before the heavy lifting begins.

FULL-BODY WORKOUT SAMPLE

Exercise	Sets	Reps	Page
1 Squat	3	10-12	112
2 Romanian deadlift	3	10-12	126
3 Pull-up	3	To failure	80
4 Bench press	3	10-12	94
5 Bent-over row	3	10-12	74
6 Seated dumb-bell shoulder press	3	10-12	138
7 Cable low-to-high woodchop	2	10 each side	159
8 Tuck and crunch	3	15-20	51

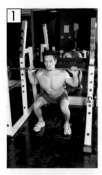
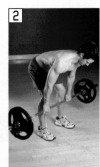
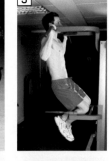
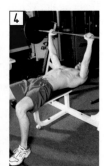
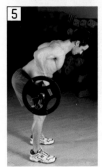
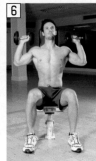
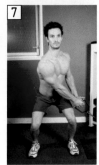
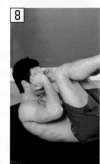

Sample Workout 2
Muscle-focus workout

If you hang around gyms for any length of time – preferably not lurking outside the ladies' changing rooms – you're sure to hear people talking about 'splits'. This simply describes how they divide up their training plans, and it's often done by body part. A typical weekly split might be: Monday, chest and triceps; Tuesday, back and biceps, Wednesday, rest; Thursday, legs; Friday, shoulders; Saturday, rest; Sunday, abs.

By focusing on a particular part of the body you can guarantee that you have trained the target muscles to the max, and then you can let them rest for a full week before hitting them again. The downside of this approach is that you can spend a lot of time working on relatively small muscles, so you're unlikely to gain as much overall muscle mass as you might have gained had you stuck to your full-body workout.

ARRANGING YOUR WORKOUT
When you give a full session to one body part, you need to think carefully about the order in which you perform your exercises. If you order your exercises correctly you'll get the best effect without over-training the muscles, as this can lead to injury. Start by doing light exercises that will warm up the joint, then move onto the big mass-moving exercises that will provide the muscle gains, and end with isolation (single-joint) moves that will take the target muscle to exhaustion. Also make sure that you keep mixing up the angles and directions from which you attack the muscle, as this will ensure you get balanced gains.

MUSCLE-FOCUS WORKOUT SAMPLE: SHOULDERS

Exercise	Sets	Reps	Page
1 Internal cable rotation	1	15-20 each side	149
2 External cable rotation	1	15-20 each side	149
3 Hang clean	2	8-10	156
4 Push press	4	10-12	137
5 High cable reverse flye	3	10-12	145
6 Lateral raise	3	10-12	142

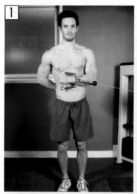
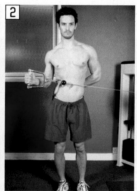
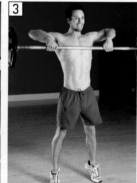
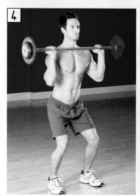
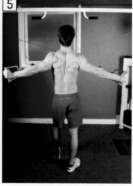
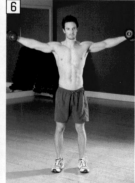

Sample Workout 3

Super-circuits

When time is short and your main goals are to burn some fat and improve your fitness, the super-circuit is a great option. You do different exercises back-to-back with no rest in between. This keeps your work rate high and forces your heart to pump blood to different parts of your body, giving you a strong cardiovascular workout as well as a muscular one.

This can be tiring, so keep the weights light, then you won't burn out too quickly. And you won't risk injury by trying to lift heavy weights when your body is in a state of exhaustion. Super-circuits aren't the best way to build bigger muscles, but they will help you look lean and defined.

ARRANGING YOUR WORKOUT

For super-circuits to be effective you need to move from one exercise to the next with minimum rest in between, so you don't want to find yourself queuing for equipment in the gym. An easy way around this is to build your workout around a single item of kit, say dumb-bells, and find a corner of the gym where you won't be disturbed. Keep the work rate high but don't perform the reps so quickly that you compromise good form.

Try to target as many different muscle groups as possible during the circuit, and switch between upper- and lower-body moves to make your heart work harder. Also, ensure you have a good blend of pushing, pulling, lunging, bending and rotational moves to keep your workout balanced throughout.

Once you've finished one circuit, take a rest of three to four minutes and then start again. The fitter you get, the more circuits you'll be able to do.

SUPER-CIRCUIT SAMPLE: DUMB-BELLS

Exercise	Sets	Reps	Page
1 Dumb-bell lateral lunge and touch	1	10 each side	123
2 Rotating squat press	1	10 each side	141
3 Bent-over flye	1	10	75
4 Lunge to press	1	10 each side	160
5 T press-up	1	10 each side	104
6 Woodchop	1	10 each side	158
7 Squat thrust	1	10	69

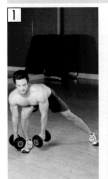
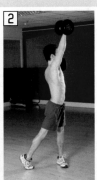
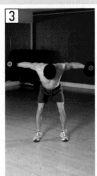
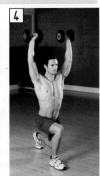

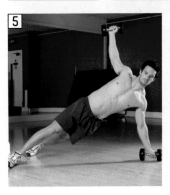
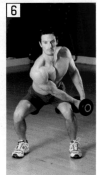
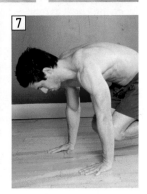

Sample Workout 4

Superset workout

The term superset simply refers to when you perform two exercises back-to-back with no rest in between. Once you've finished both exercises you rest and then perform the superset again – just as you would if you were performing normal sets. The idea is that you can place your muscles under tension for longer without increasing the length of your workout, and unlike a super-circuit you can afford to go heavy on each exercise, making this an effective muscle-building technique.

Any two exercises together can be a superset, but the most popular form of this training is to perform what's known as an 'antagonistic superset'. This means that each exercise is the muscular opposite of the other. So for example, if you were to do a bench press (which works your chest) and follow this immediately by a bent-over row (which works your back) then this would be an antagonistic superset.

The advantage of antagonistic supersets is that one muscle group gets to rest while you work the other, and you guarantee balanced results by giving equal attention to opposing muscle groups.

ARRANGING YOUR WORKOUT
For each exercise, try to imagine its polar opposite, so if you do one exercise that works your quads you need to pair it with one that works your hamstrings. Biceps exercises should be paired with triceps exercises, and so on.

After each superset rest for a couple of minutes before repeating.

SUPERSET WORKOUT SAMPLE

Exercise		Sets	Reps	Page
Superset 1	Incline bench press	3	10-12	98
	Bent-over row		10-12	74
Superset 2	Cross-grip front squat	3	10-12	117
	Stiff-legged Romanian deadlift		10-12	127
Superset 3	EZ-bar curl	3	10-12	19
	EZ-bar overhead triceps extension		10-12	37
Superset 4	Weighted crunch	3	10-12	49
	Swiss ball back extension		10-12	89

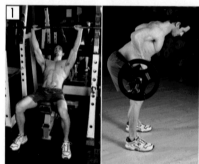
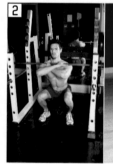
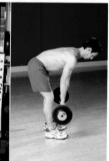
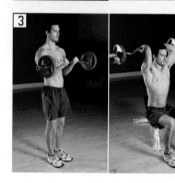
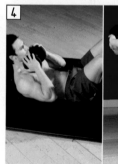
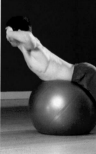

Sample Workout 5
Drop set workout

Y ou'll be pleased to learn that a drop set has nothing to do with dropping heavy dumb-bells on your foot. Drop set simply refers to a training method whereby you perform a standard set of reps to failure. Then once you've reached that point you immediately drop the weight by about 15-20 per cent and crank out a few more reps until you hit failure again. As soon as you do, you drop the weight by 15-20 per cent again and do more reps, and so on.

This is an excellent way to shock your muscles into more growth. However drop sets can place a great deal of stress on your body so you shouldn't overuse this method or you will soon suffer from over-training. You should only use drop sets on the last set of any exercise and only do it once or twice per muscle group per session. You should also make sure you leave a few weeks between drop set workouts to let your body recover.

ARRANGING YOUR WORKOUT
A training partner is useful when you're performing drop sets because he or she can do the job of dropping the weights for you. A spotter (a person who stops you from dropping a barbell on your head during bench presses) can strip weights from the bar quickly and save you time between reps.

Pick exercises in your workout that will suit drop sets best. Compound exercises that use a lot of muscle fibres are best, but make sure you can maintain perfect form for the exercise even when your muscles are fully exhausted.

DROP SET WORKOUT SAMPLE: CHEST & TRICEPS

Exercise	Sets	Reps	Page
1 Alternating jump press-up	3	10	105
2 Bench press	3 (last set drop set)	10-12	94
3 Cable crossover	2	10-12	103
4 Bench dip	3	10	28
5 Triceps press down	3 (last set drop set)	10-12	40
6 Unilateral wall press-up	2	10	33

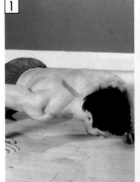
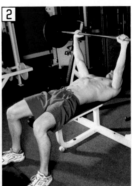
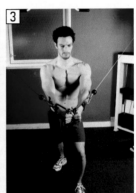
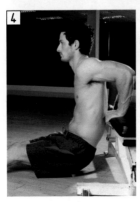
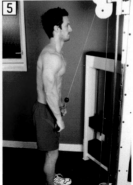
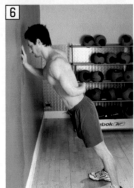

Sample Workout 6

Post-exhaustion workout

All weight-training exercises are either a compound or an isolation move. Put another way, some exercises use several muscle groups at once, while others target one muscle group specifically. With post-exhaustion training the trick is to pair compound with isolation moves to stimulate muscle growth.

The compound move should always come first. This gets your target muscle pumped by moving heavy weights, aided by other muscle groups. Then you can move on to the isolation move, which uses lighter weights but targets the muscle directly with no interference from other muscle groups. For example, if you were training your chest, you might do sets of bench presses (compound move: your chest muscles are aided by your shoulders and triceps) and follow them with sets of dumb-bell flyes (isolation move: targets your pecs exclusively). The result is that your pecs get the best chance for growth because they have moved heavy weights, followed quickly by being taken to full exhaustion by the isolation move.

ARRANGING YOUR WORKOUT

For each body part pick a compound exercise and follow it with an isolation move. Don't be tempted to do it the other way round, even if you've heard trainers talk about 'pre-exhaustion' techniques. If you do the isolation move first, there's a risk that your target muscle will be too tired to handle the heavy weights of the compound move and will transfer the strain onto the supporting muscles, which can easily become injured.

POST-EXHAUSTION WORKOUT SAMPLE

Exercise	Sets	Reps	Page
1 Squat	3	10-12	112
2 One-leg Smith squat	2	10-12 each leg	115
3 Bench press	3	10-12	94
4 Dumb-bell flye	3	10-12	102
5 Romanian deadlift	3	10-12	126
6 Swiss ball leg curl	3	10	128
7 Cable row	3	10-12	76
8 Bent-over flye	3	10-12	75

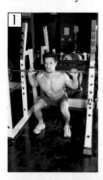
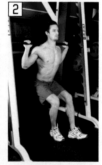
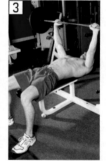
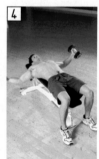
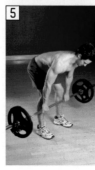
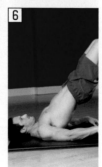
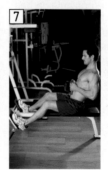
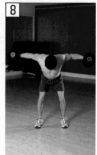

Sample Workout 7

Core-stability workout

The importance of core training has increased dramatically in recent years as more fitness coaches come to understand the vital role that the core muscles play in all areas of physical performance.

Your core – the muscles around your midriff, including your abdominals and lower back – are the link between your upper and lower body. Any movement that uses the whole body requires a strong core to transfer power between the upper and lower halves, and to stabilise your spine when performing dynamic moves. Whether you are running, cycling, power lifting, playing tennis, kicking a football or simply picking up your baby from his cot, your core muscles are hard at work keeping you upright. Weak core muscles are often the cause of lower-back pain and can result in poor posture – and who wants to look like a teenager all their life?

ARRANGING YOUR WORKOUT
Many men spend hours in the gym working on their abdominals to get that all-important washboard stomach, but when it comes to core training equal emphasis needs to be placed on the muscles at the sides and back of your midriff to get the greatest possible benefit.

Attack your core muscles from several different angles and include rotational moves to give your core a thorough workout. Start with moves that place the greatest weight on your core, such as compound lifts, and end with bodyweight exercises that won't risk injuring your tired muscles.

CORE-STABILITY WORKOUT SAMPLE

Exercise	Sets	Reps	Page
1 Deadlift	3	10-12	154
2 Split squat to one-arm row	2	10-12 each arm	79
3 Swiss ball crunch	2	15	49
4 Swiss ball back extension	2	15	89
5 Swiss ball oblique crunch	2	15 each side	53
6 Two-point box	2	15 each side	88
7 Swiss ball Russian twist	2	15 each side	67
8 Plank	1	Hold as long as possible	58

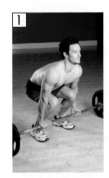
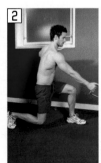
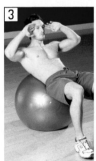
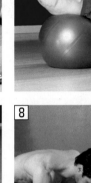
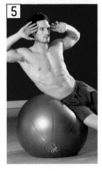
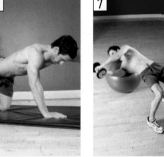
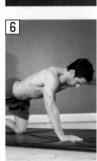

Tips on training

A few things to keep in mind whenever you do a workout

1 KEEP YOUR CORE TIGHT
Before any heavy lift, tighten your core muscles – the ones around your midriff – to protect your lower back from injury. Imagine someone is going to punch you in the stomach and brace your abs. Now hold it like that for the duration of the lift.

2 WATCH YOUR SPEED
Each set of each exercise should take you around 40 seconds to complete. Any faster and you're not putting your muscles under tension long enough to get good results. Therefore, each rep should take three or four seconds. Make the lowering (eccentric) portion of the lift slow and controlled, and then move powerfully through the exertion (concentric) part of the lift.

3 DON'T FORGET TO BREATHE
Never hold your breath during a heavy lift. Instead the general rule is to breathe in as you lower the weight, and breathe out through pursed lips as you lift the weight.

4 GET SOME BALANCE
Is one side of your body stronger than the other? It's fairly common for right-handed men to have a stronger right arm, and if you always stick to

barbell moves your right side will end up doing most of the work, so be sure to introduce unilateral (one-sided) moves into your workouts to balance out your strength gains.

5 PICK YOUR WEIGHT
The correct weight is the one that allows you to complete all the reps of your set with perfect form, but no more. When you first begin training you'll need a bit of trial and error to determine the weights that suit you. Err on the light side and build up, not the other way round. Leave your ego at the door – there's no sadder sight than a man struggling to lift weights that are plainly too heavy for him.

6 MAKE YOUR WORKOUTS PROGRESSIVE
Aim to increase the resistance you use for an exercise by around 10 per cent every three or four weeks. This will ensure that your muscles get the stimulation they need to grow. If the weights don't get bigger then neither will your muscles.

7 MIND YOUR MANNERS
There are a few unwritten rules of gym etiquette that you should follow if you don't want to be ostracised by your fellow gym members. Always

replace dumb-bells and weight plates on their racks after you've used them. Never hog a machine or a piece of equipment. Wipe your sweat off any equipment after you've used it. Don't trail water from the showers into the changing rooms. And don't grunt like a constipated baboon during lifts (that's less of a rule, more a pet-hate of ours).

8 STAY HYDRATED
Most gyms provide water, but a sensible move is to take a bottle with you so you can sip from it every few minutes to keep your water levels topped up. If you wait until you're thirsty before drinking, the chances are you're already dehydrated and your performance will suffer as a result.

9 EAT STRAIGHT AFTER YOUR WORKOUT
The 45 minutes immediately after you finish your last rep are vital for getting muscle-replenishing nutrients into your body, so take a snack with you to the gym. A mixture of high-GI carbohydrates, fast-acting protein and antioxidants is best. See the section on food (p181) for what to eat.

10 MIX IT UP
Your body is very clever – it quickly adapts to any stresses placed

upon it so that it can perform the actions more efficiently. What that means is that if you always do the same workout your body will adapt to it and stop growing new muscle. Keep altering your workout every few weeks, even if that simply means using different items of equipment, changing the angle on your bench, or altering the order you perform the exercises in. Change is good for your muscles.

11 GET YOUR REST

Your muscles don't grow while you're working out in the gym. They grow when they are recovering afterwards. That's why you shouldn't train the same muscle groups two days in a row. If you do they won't have had time to repair themselves from the first workout by the time you hit them again. If you want more muscle, always take rest days and make sure you get enough sleep.

12 ENJOY IT

The plan you stick with is the plan you enjoy. If training seems like a chore then it's unlikely you'll keep it up, so look for ways of making it fun. Put your favourite music on, do activities you enjoy, and get your mates involved – the rivalry can be motivational as well as good fun.

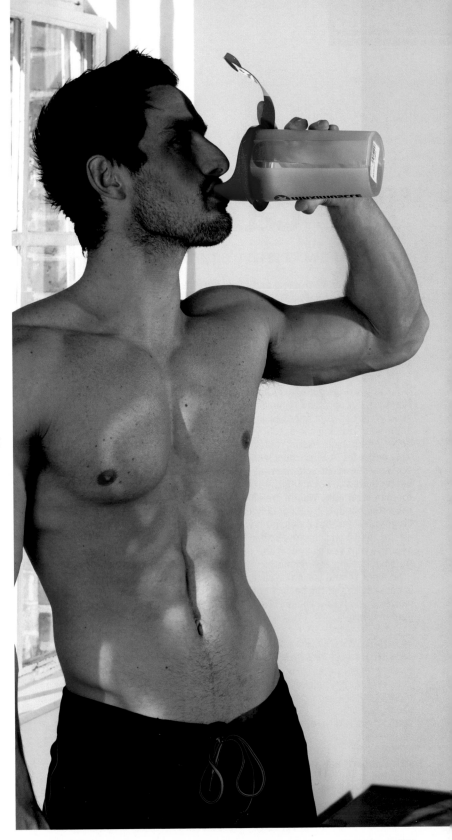

The cardio question

Should you do weights *and* cardio training? The answer is yes, but...

Generally weight training and cardio training don't get on. They look different, they behave differently, they achieve different results. They glower at each other across the gym and make snippy remarks about how the other one isn't 'real fitness'.

The problem is that cardio training, while improving your heart and lung function, doesn't tend to have a good effect on your muscles. In fact endurance training can actually break down your muscle tissue, replacing your bulky fast-twitch muscles with scrawny slow-twitch fibres that are better suited to pounding the streets for mile after mile. Weight training, on the other hand, is great for building bigger muscles, but it doesn't have all the health and cardiovascular benefits that you can get from running, cycling or swimming.

So what should you do? Well, it is possible to get the best of both worlds if you follow these three golden rules:

1 DON'T MIX CARDIO AND WEIGHTS ON THE SAME DAY

If your primary goal is to build new muscle mass it's best to keep your weights sessions and cardio sessions separate. Some body builders eschew cardio training altogether, arguing that cardio has a catabolic effect on muscle (it breaks down muscle tissue) and that lifting weights provides a sufficient fat-burning and heart-pumping effect to maintain good health. However, most fitness trainers would agree that you can't beat cardiovascular training

for torching unwanted calories and improving health – it's simply a case of knowing how to combine it effectively with your muscle-building goals.

Doing cardio immediately before doing a weights session will leave you feeling tired and will lead to a poor lifting performance. Doing cardio immediately after a weights session can mean you negate the muscle-building effects you've just achieved. The answer is to do them on separate days. That way your muscles have had time to recover before you lace up your running shoes and hit the streets.

Of course, if your primary goal is fat loss, then mixing cardio exercise and weights can be beneficial, but only if you follow rule two:

2 KEEP IT SHORT AND INTENSE

When you begin a run (or any other cardio activity) your body uses energy from your fat supplies and from the food you eat. After about 45 minutes of exercise it then switches to take energy from your muscles, and soon it starts to break down your muscle tissue to keep you going as you plod along the pavement. So much for all that hard work you put in lifting weights. But there is a way you can avoid this, and that, if you haven't guessed it already, is to keep your cardio sessions to under 45 minutes.

You can get all the benefits of a long run in a short time by increasing the intensity of your exercise, and the best way to do this is with intervals. An interval session is when you do short bursts of intense exercise interspersed

with recovery periods, so a 20-minute interval session might look like this:

20-MINUTE INTERVAL SESSION

5 minutes	**Slow warm-up run**
1 minute	**Run at 80% of**
	maximum effort (ME)
2 minutes	**Run at 40% of ME**
1 minute	**Run at 80% of ME**
2 minutes	**Run at 40% of ME**
1 minute	**Run at 80% of ME**
2 minutes	**Run at 40% of ME**
1 minute	**Run at 80% of ME**
5 minutes	**Slow warm-down run**

Intervals have been proven to be more effective than steady-state running at burning fat, raising your metabolism and improving cardiovascular health. Their other benefit is that they will have minimal impact on your hard-won muscle.

As your fitness improves you can increase the duration of the intense portions of your intervals, and shorten the time you take on the recovery periods. This makes the session tougher without it lasting any longer.

3 KEEP EATING

Good nutrition is vital to achieving the body you want. If you are doing both weight training and cardio it becomes even more important because you need to fuel your exertions in the cardio sessions and still have enough calories to build the muscle you've trained so hard for.

To find out what foods you need to eat and how much turn to p181.

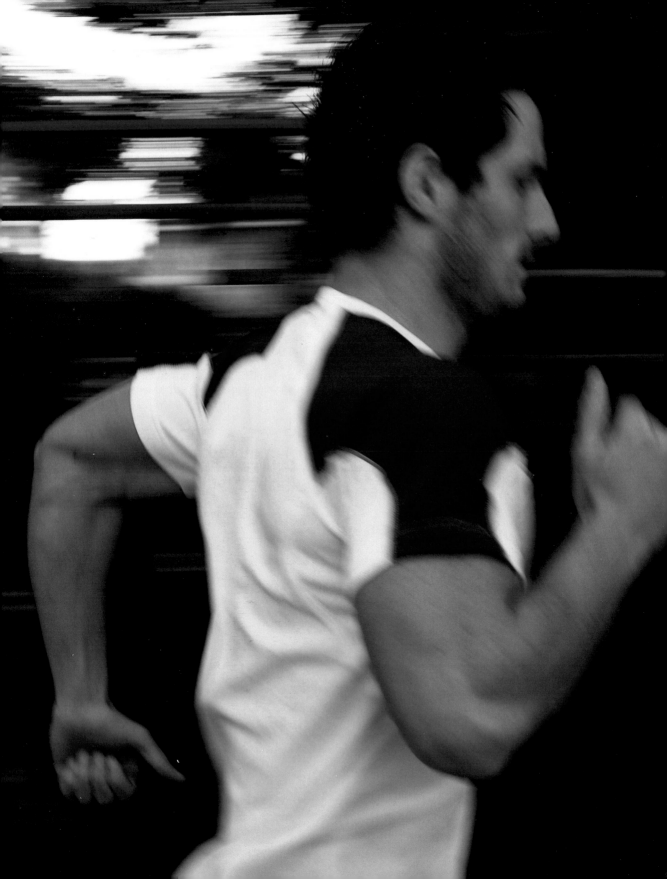

Chart your progress

You'll stick with your training plan better if you keep track of your workouts

We've already mentioned the importance of having a plan when you enter the gym. If you just wander from machine to machine with no real idea of what you are trying to achieve, then the result will be that you achieve very little. But if you know exactly which exercises you want to do – and why – then your workout will be more effective and more enjoyable.

Keeping a log is the easiest way to plan your workouts and track your progress. Once you've written down the exercises you intend to do, it automatically focuses your mind and motivates you to train hard in the gym, and you'll be able to see your achievements there in black and white. It's very gratifying to look back at old training logs and realise just how much more you are lifting than when you started.

USING A TRAINING LOG

On the opposite page we've given you a template you can use for your training log. Take it to work and photocopy it several times when the boss isn't looking then use the pages to make yourself a long-term training logbook. Before every workout, write the details of what you intend to do in the spaces, taking note of the weights you have used previously so that you can aim to beat your personal bests all the time. Then, once you've completed your workout, tick the 'done' boxes and add any notes you think might be helpful in your next workout.

The template doesn't take into account such things as supersets or drop sets, but you can find your own way of personalising your log – after all, you are the only person who is going to look at it, so your log only has to make sense to you. Just try not to make it too complicated.

Here we've given you an example of how you might fill in your log for one workout. Stick with your training log and you'll stick with your training.

Date 15th May	Workout Chest & Triceps				
Warm up 10 mins rower + dynamic stretches				(tick when done)	☑
Exercise	Sets	Reps	Weight		
1 Press up	2	15-20	—		☑
2 Bent over row	1	15-20	30kg		☑
3 Bench press	3	10-12	45kg		☑
4 Dumb-bell flye	3	10-12	12kg		☑
5 Bench dip	3	12-15	—		☑
6 Seated one arm overhead tri extension	2	10-12 each arm	10kg		☑
7 Rope press down	3	10-12	Set pin at plate 4		☑
8					☐
9					☐
10					☐
Warm down and stretch 10 mins crosstrainer + stretches					☐
Cardio —					
Notes Aim to increase bench press weight to 50kg at next session.					

Date	Workout

Warm up			(tick when done) ☐

Exercise	**Sets**	**Reps**	**Weight**	
1				☐
2				☐
3				☐
4				☐
5				☐
6				☐
7				☐
8				☐
9				☐
10				☐

Warm down and stretch	☐

Cardio

Notes

Eat for muscle

Training is only half the game – the other half takes place in the kitchen

All the weight training in the world will come to nothing without the correct nutrition to back it up. Muscles need calories to grow. They also need the right combinations of carbohydrates for energy, protein for muscle repair and fats to protect joints and improve metabolism. Plus your diet needs to include a good range of vitamins and minerals as these will help protect your body from the ravages of intense training.

When you exercise, your body produces 'free radicals' that can cause muscle soreness and general discomfort (and if left unchecked can even lead to heart disease or cancer) so a diet rich in antioxidants is also recommended for people who do a lot of training. Antioxidants are enzymes and nutrients that can fight free radicals and they are found in a range of vegetables, fruits, seeds, nuts, grains and even red wine.

GET THE BASICS RIGHT
Nutrition for weight training is a subject that could easily fill a whole book, and unfortunately there isn't the space in this guide to cover it in detail. However, over the next two pages we have given you the golden rules for eating to gain muscle, and on p184 you'll find a sample meal plan that provides the right combination of carbs, protein, fats and antioxidants to get the best results from your training. We're not suggesting that you rigidly stick to the menus week in, week out. Rather you should use it as a template for creating your own meal plans incorporating as wide a range of different foods as you can. Believe us our body will thank you for it.

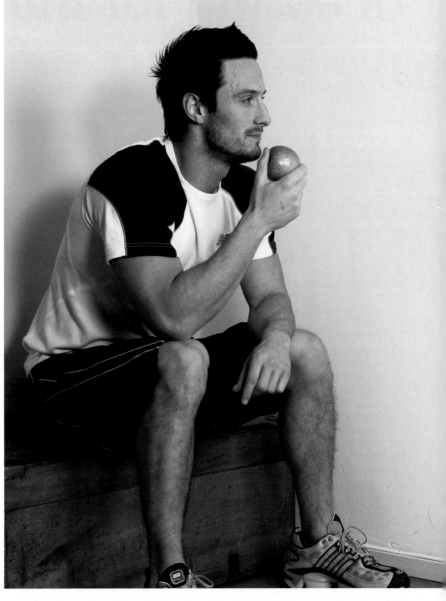

The six golden rules of eating for muscle

1 INCREASE YOUR CALORIE INTAKE

The maths is fairly simple. If you eat fewer calories each day than you burn off through activity, you will lose weight. If you eat more, you'll gain weight. And if you eat more of the right things combined with a proper weight training strategy, you'll gain the weight as muscle rather than fat.

The average man needs around 2,500 calories a day just to stay at the same weight, so consider increasing this to around 3,000 calories a day. Some of that extra will be burned off during your workouts, but the rest will go to growing your muscles, and you should see a steady weight gain of around 1kg a month depending on your natural body type.

2 GET THE BALANCE RIGHT

Nearly all your calories come from a combination of carbohydrate, protein and fats.

Carbohydrates are vital to provide the muscle glycogen that fuels your workouts and should make up about 60 per cent of your total calorie intake, which equates to around 450g of carbohydrates a day if your total calorie intake is 3,000.

Protein is required to grow new tissue in your body and is therefore of special interest to anyone building muscle. However, don't believe the gym myth that more protein equals more muscle. For most men anything over 180g of protein a day is largely useless. The optimum intake of protein for muscle-gainers is between 1.5g and 2g of protein per kilogram of bodyweight. So, if you weigh 80kg you'll require 120g-160g of protein a day, which will make up around 20 per cent of your daily 3,000 calories.

Fat makes up the final 20 per cent of your calories. Fats can help you absorb vitamins, improve athletic performance and protect joints and tendons from injury. However fat is very energy-dense, containing nine calories per gram compared to four calories for carbs and protein, so your daily 600 calories of fat weighs just 67g.

3 EAT THE RIGHT STUFF

The simplest rule when deciding what to eat is: keep it natural. Processed foods – biscuits, cakes, ready meals, fizzy drinks, crisps – tend to be high on calories but low on essential nutrients, so they are poor at fuelling workouts and rebuilding muscle but good at making you fat and sapping your energy reserves.

Carbohydrates come in many different forms, and many studies have looked at which carbs are best for fuelling and recovering from workouts. To keep things simple aim to make the majority of your carbs unrefined, unprocessed, low on the glycaemic index and high in fibre. This includes wholemeal bread and pasta, oats, beans, fruit and vegetables. These will release energy slowly and regulate your blood-sugar levels, ensuring you always have enough stored glycogen in your muscles for an energetic workout.

Protein-rich foods include lean meat, fish, eggs, dairy produce and soya. Lower quality protein can also be found in nuts, seeds and beans. Aim to eat a wide variety of protein-rich foods to ensure you get the full range of muscle-building amino acids, but be wary of taking in too much saturated fat, such as that found in poor cuts of red meat and dairy items.

Fats come in four forms: saturates, found in meat and dairy products; monounsaturates, found in olive oil, nuts and seeds; polyunsaturates, found in vegetable oils and oily fish; and trans fats, which are produced by hydrogenating oils to make a solid fat used in cakes, biscuits and margarine. The simple rule here is to keep saturates and trans fats to an absolute minimum, as they can increase the risk of heart disease, and stock up on monounsaturates and polyunsaturates, especially the omega 3 and omega 6 varieties. Omega 3 fats, as found in oily fish such as mackerel, tuna and sardines, have been proven to aid strength and aerobic training and protect the body from injuries.

4 TIME YOUR MEALS

When your goal is bigger muscles, the most important time to eat is immediately after your workout. This is when your muscles have used up vital glycogen stores and are crying out for replenishment. Aim to eat a high-carbohydrate snack mixed with some protein within 45 minutes of finishing your last rep in the gym. Something like a bagel with cream cheese is perfect, or a tuna and pasta salad.

For the rest of the day, eat small meals at regular intervals of two or three hours, with the aim of having some protein with every meal. This way you keep your glycogen levels topped up and prevent your body from breaking down the proteins that you need for muscle rebuilding.

5 MORE WATER, LESS BOOZE

It goes without saying that if you sweat a lot in the gym you're going to need to replace that fluid with water. The trick is to ensure that you hydrate yourself before you get thirsty, not afterwards. Dehydration will impact on your performance in the gym and can affect the way your body stores fat and repairs muscle owing to poor organ function. Take a water bottle with you to the gym and sip from it every few minutes rather than glugging it all down in one go (which will just make you want to pee more). Over the course of a day you should aim to take in about three litres of water in total.

Booze, on the other hand, you can do without. Alcohol can have a catabolic effect on your muscles, meaning it prevents them from developing properly. If you are serious about gaining muscle mass, keep your sessions in the pub to a minimum.

6 THE SUPPLEMENT QUESTION

Should you or shouldn't you take nutritional supplements? The answer is that they shouldn't be seen as a alternative to a good diet. Despite the claims of some protein powders or of fat-burning pills, if you are eating properly and following the rules we've outlined above, there really is no need to take supplements, especially as these can prove to be expensive.

That said, if you find you're having a problem consuming the necessary calories each day, meal-replacement drinks are an easy way to get extra protein and carbs without unwanted fat. Also, people who do a lot of exercise can often need extra vitamins C and E, so a supplement of these can be handy if you struggle to get enough in your regular diet.

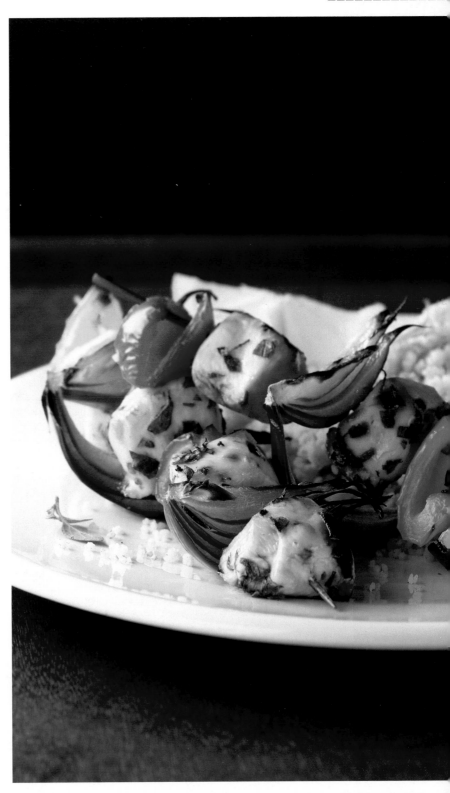

Muscle meals

This plan shows you the kinds of foods you should be eating every day to add lean muscle mass

	MON	TUE	WED	THU	FRI
Breakfast	45g oats with 300ml skimmed milk, 1tsp honey and 25g whey protein.	Two pieces of French toast made with 1 egg, 1 pint milk and 2tsp cinnamon and nutmeg.	4 scrambled egg whites on 2 slices of wholemeal toast. 1 grapefruit.	2 slices French toast made with 1 egg, 1 pint milk and 2tsp cinnamon and nutmeg.	Smoothie with 25g whey protein, 300ml skimmed milk, 100g strawberries, ½ banana and 1tsp flaxseed oil.
Snack	90g sardines on 2 slices of wholemeal toast. Orange juice.	120g low-fat yoghurt with blueberries, honey and oats. 1 protein bar.	Mixed nuts, raisins and cranberries.	1 mashed banana on 1 slice of wholemeal toast. 1 protein bar.	1 low-fat yoghurt with blueberries, oats and honey.
Lunch	Medium jacket potato with tuna, baked beans and grated cheese.	Turkey and cranberry sandwich on wholemeal bread. 1 pear.	Turkey and cheese salad sandwich on a wholemeal roll. 1 pear.	Turkey salad sandwich on wholemeal bread. 1 apple.	Medium jacket potato with baked beans and cottage cheese.
Snack	Smoothie with 25g whey protein, 80g raspberries, 80g blueberries and 50g blackberries, blended with water.	Smoothie with 25g whey protein, 300ml skimmed milk, 100g strawberries, ½ banana and 1tsp flaxseed oil.	Smoothie with 24g whey protein, 80g raspberries, 80g blueberries and 50g blackberries, blended with water.	Mixed nuts, raisins and cranberries with cottage cheese.	140g grilled chicken and beetroot.
Dinner	200g chicken and vegetable stir-fry with red and green peppers, sesame seeds and oil.	70g wholemeal pasta and 100g lean minced beef with tomato sauce and a chopped onion.	2 chicken breasts, diced and stir-fried with ½ onion, 1 red pepper and 1 clove of garlic, then sautéed in canned tomatoes and chicken stock. 70g basmati rice. 1 portion of steamed broccoli.	1 grilled salmon fillet served with stir-fried pak choi, red peppers and almonds.	120g tuna steak with stir-fried broccoli, green beans and spinach with sesame seeds and oil. 70g brown rice.
Snack	120g low-fat yoghurt with strawberries.	100g cottage cheese and pineapple.	Smoothie with 25g protein, 300ml skimmed milk, 50g blueberries, 50g blackberries ½ banana.	Smoothie with 25g protein, 300ml skimmed milk, 50g blueberries, 50g blackberries ½ banana.	Smoothie with 25g whey protein, 80g raspberries, 80g blueberries and 50g blackberries, blended with water.
Total calories	2,876	2,823	2,847	2,825	2,910

SAT	SUN
445g oats with 300ml skimmed milk, 1tsp of honey and 25g whey protein.	3 scrambled eggs on 2 slices of wholemeal toast. 1 grapefruit. Orange juice.
1 mashed banana on 2 slices of wholemeal toast.	1 mashed banana with 2tbsp peanut butter on wholemeal toast.
Turkey and cheese salad sandwich on wholemeal bread. 1 apple.	Medium jacket potato with baked beans and cottage cheese.
1 can of tuna with beetroot. 1 low-fat yoghurt.	Smoothie with 25g whey protein, 80g raspberries, 80g blueberries and 50g blackberries, blended with water. 30g brazil nuts.
120g fillet steak with medium jacket potato, grilled tomato and spinach.	Roast lamb with 100g new potatoes and mixed vegetables.
Smoothie with 25g whey protein, 300ml skimmed milk, 100g strawberries, ½ banana and 1tsp flaxseed oil.	Smoothie with 25g whey protein, 300ml skimmed milk, 100g strawberries, ½ banana and 1tsp flaxseed oil.
2,976	2,991

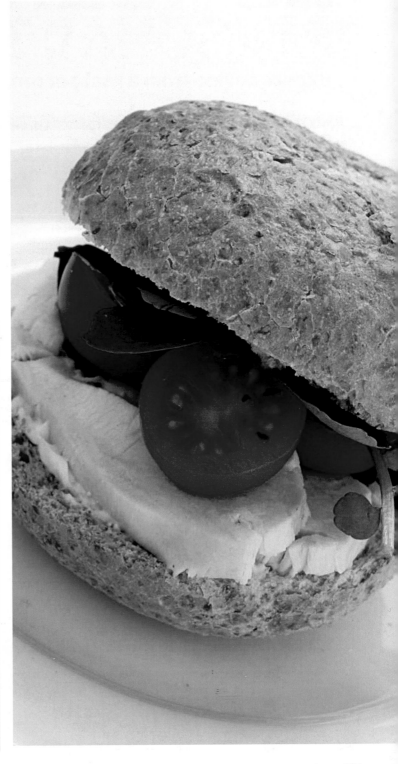

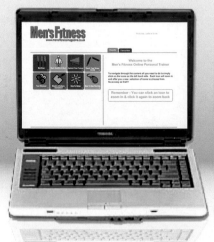
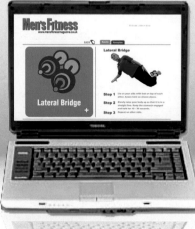
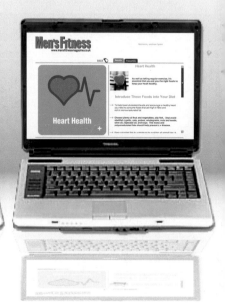
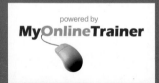